HEMPHILL'S

HERBS
FOR
HEALTH

John and Rosemary
HEMPHILL

First published 1985 by Lansdowne Press, Sydney
a division of RPLA Pty Limited
176 South Creek Road, Dee Why West, N.S.W., Australia, 2099.

© Copyright John and Rosemary Hemphill

First published in the UK by Blandford Press
Link House, West Street, Poole, Dorset

Distributed in the United States by
Sterling Publishing Co. Inc.,
2 Park Avenue, New York, NY 10016

ISBN 0 7137 1763 7

Typeset in Australia by Deblaere Typesetting Pty Ltd
Printed in Hong Kong by Everbest Printing Co. Ltd

HEMPHILL'S

HERBS
FOR
HEALTH

John and Rosemary
HEMPHILL

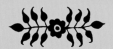

BLANDFORD PRESS
POOLE   DORSET

For Gwennyth and George

ACKNOWLEDGEMENTS

We would like to express our sincere thanks and appreciation for the support and genuine interest of the staff at Lansdowne Press, both in Australia and in England, before, and during the writing of this book. In Australia the Publisher, Anne Wilson, has given us kind encouragement; Christine Alderton's illustrations have portrayed with delicacy the feeling we wished to convey in the writing; Susan Tomnay, the Managing Editor, has unstintingly given sound advice and inspiration, and Doreen Grézoux has edited the work with sensitivity. Carole Saunders and Amelia Thorpe from the London office have warmed our hearts with their enthusiasm.

We are grateful to Clare Wilmot of the Triad Clinic for allowing us to draw on her skilled knowledge of herbal medicine, which was of great assistance in authenticating some of our research.

CONTENTS

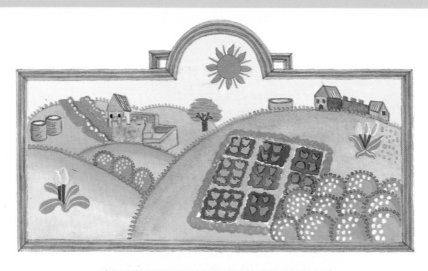

HISTORY OF HERBS

The history and romance of herbs is wreathed in the dim mists of time to intrigue and enchant us. Herbs are mentioned in the Bible many times in both the Old and New Testaments. They also appear in Greek mythology, fennel being an example. Legend has it that the god Prometheus went up to heaven holding a hollow fennel stalk in which he concealed some of the sun's fire to bring back to earth for man's use.

From the time the written word was set down on papyrus, or incised into wax or stone tablets, the use of herbs in countless different ways was reported. Most of our ancestors' knowledge came from pure instinct, as a result of living close to nature, and it is interesting to learn that today's scientists are proving much of this lore to be correct. Many of these old methods of healing are gaining new

followers and are a continuing part of natural therapeutics.

The ancient Egyptians and Greeks were the first people known to write down in technical terms their knowledge of herbs, following their scholarly, systematic observations of plant life. Indian and Asian civilisations, which were very advanced at an early time, also knew the value of plants that grew on their continents.

In Egypt, herbs were used extensively about 2700 B.C. They grew abundantly in the rich soil by the River Nile and were concocted into potions and ointments and, together with rare and exotic spices, were used for embalming the dead. Medical schools began to flourish in Egypt and it is thought that the Greek physician Hippocrates was a student at one of these schools. Another great Greek physician, Dioscorides, who lived during the reign of Nero, was the author of a herbal materia medica, and it is said that for a thousand years afterwards, doctors in the known world used his remedies for healing the sick.

Pliny the Elder (A.D. 23–79), who perished during the eruption of Vesuvius which destroyed Pompeii, and his nephew, known as Pliny the Younger (A.D. 62c–113), were Roman historians who left detailed records of life in their times, including many treatises on herbs; however, it is thought that the elder Pliny was the author of the works on herbs. He is still quoted today in herbal encyclopedias.

At historical Ephesus, herbs can be seen growing abundantly and flowering amongst fallen columns and between paving stones; there is even a small basil plant flourishing bravely in brown, hard, inhospitable ground. This landlocked city of white marble ruins, extensive and preserved enough to captivate the imagination forever, lies glittering in the sunlight as it has done for several thousand years. It was once a seaport where, legend says,

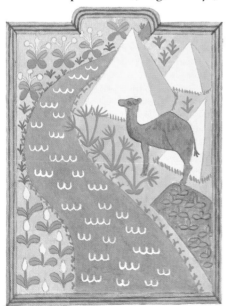

Antony and Cleopatra disembarked from their vessel and walked along the lovely streets. Later St Paul visited Ephesus, and it is claimed that the Virgin Mary spent the last years of her life nearby. She was taken there by St John after the Crucifixion for protection.

In Crete, among the green slopes of Knossos, stepping through some of the partially restored and originally enormous Minoan Palace, where Theseus slew the fearsome Minotaur in the Labyrinth, is an exquisite wall painting of an immensely elegant azure-blue monkey, sitting with one "hand" poised above a stylised saffron flower. Apparently monkeys were trained to pluck the orange stigmas from the heart of the saffron crocus because of their dexterous fingers and very long nails. Saffron was valued for the delicate flavour and colour it gave to food (it is highly prized today for the same reason), and its golden-yellow dye was used to colour cloth and tint the hair.

In early England it is believed that there were ancient herbal writings which were destroyed during the Danish invasions. Old manuscripts on the subject, now in safe-keeping in Britain, are the 10th century *Leech Book of Bald* and the Saxon translations of the *Herbarium of Apuleius*. These documents bear out the knowledge that the use of herbs dated from the earliest times. Certain plants were an essential ingredient in charms, spells and ceremonies, as well as in remedies, and some herbs in particular were believed to ward off treacherous water elves, "the flying venom", trolls and evil spirits. Other herbs were used in remedies, in food, and for dyeing.

When the conquering Romans came to Britain and settled for two hundred years or so, they brought with them the herbs that were essential in their food and medicines. We think of these plants today as being indigenous to Britain but they are actually native to the Mediterranean. Some of these are oregano, marjoram, thyme, sage, rosemary, balm, bay trees, fennel, savory and mint.

Herbs were continually being introduced by newcomers: the invading Normans would have seen to it that their diet in a new land still contained their favourite herbs and that their medicine boxes held the "physics" that they knew were effective. Various foreign princesses who became queens of England were influential in importing others; the Countess of Hainault, mother of Philippa, wife of Edward III, sent her daughter a famous manuscript dealing with the virtues of herbs. People who were travelling and adventuring to other countries also found new and diverse plants to bring home.

In the Middle Ages monks cultivated herbs intensively and made many advances in their cultivation and use, discovering many more properties, which they recorded. It is well known that the first liqueurs were concocted by monks as potent medicines. A small glass (the forerunner of the liqueur glass), containing the carefully blended precious plant essences, would be administered to the patients who came to the good monks to be healed in body as well as in soul.

Later were to come other great herbalists like John Gerard (16th century), John Parkinson (17th century), and Nicholas Culpeper (17th century). Other herbalists, gardeners and gourmets have set down their own delightful and helpful observations during the following three hundred years.

Wherever the human race has traded or settled, herbs and spices have been woven into history. It is amazing to consider the ability of herbs to spread

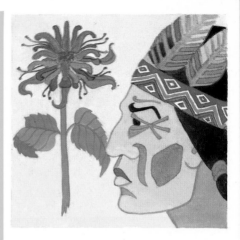

and grow in remote corners of the ancient and the modern world.

The Pilgrim Fathers took herbs with them to America. Many were already indigenous to the new land, including bergamot, used by the Oswego Indians as a curative herb. The new settlers soon found "Oswego Tea" a remedy for sore throats and colds, and its soft fragrance made a delicious herbal tea. "Johnny Appleseed", as he was called, helped spread many herbs from his home to families in the new land.

The first white settlers in Australia brought with them herb seeds to grow in a new and strange continent to use as flavouring for their food, as medicines, and to make into sweet bags and potpourri to perfume rooms and closets. Stories abound of grandmother's favourite herbal remedies and these pioneers were not afraid to experiment with some of the native Australian flora, such as ti-tree leaves, which it is said they used for making tea, the lemon-scented variety being highly favoured. People also learned much in those early days from the Aborigines. But for many years the popularity of herbs declined and those which were once in everyday use became obscure and their names strange. There are exceptions of course, like parsley, mint, sage, thyme, marjoram and chives, and in the last twenty years there has been a remarkable world-wide resurgence of interest in herbs.

The Aboriginal people knew about their own wild plants and how to apply them for various needs but most Australians know very little about these plants. However, an excellent book by A. B. and N. W. Cribb, published by Collins, called *Wild Medicine in Australia,* provides a wealth of information on a large range of native species that have been used by the Aborigines and early European settlers to treat a number of diseases.

Herbs have been defined under several different headings: physic or medicinal; flavouring or culinary; fragrant, and those used for dyeing. In many countries they grow as wild as weeds along hedgerows and wasteland. Once a weed has become useful it reaches the status of being called a herb. Physic herbs were once called "simples" because specific ones contained the effective components for remedying simple ills.

Fragrant or "sweet herbs" were those whose aromatic leaves and flowers were strewn on floors to sweeten the air as they were trodden on (and to keep away unwanted insects and vermin). They were picked and dried for a potpourri blend, for sweet bags, and for incorporating into numerous other household recipes in the still-room of the mistress of the house.

Herbs and some vegetables were also important for dyeing cloth.

"Pot herbs" were more like an early form of vegetable. They were used in cooking for the flavour and nourishment in their leaves, roots and stems.

"Salad herbs", eaten raw, were usually leafy and included many chopped-up culinary herbs.

Herbs contain their own particular properties and essences and some medicinal plants if taken in large quantities can be poisonous. If prescribed in the correct proportions and mixtures by a trained practitioner they can be quite effective. Many chemical medicines today have been derived, then synthesised, from herbs. The sedative drug Valium is a synthesised substance found in the root of the herb valerian, long esteemed for its calming and soothing effect. The pretty foxglove((*Digitalis purpurea*) is a plant which is a heart drug, and can be fatal if the leaves are eaten as a salad. A derivative of foxglove is today a chemical orthodox drug and is prescribed with safety by doctors for certain heart ailments. Medicinal plants are beyond the scope of this book, which deals mainly with culinary and salad herbs which are tasty and health-giving. When eating them, or taking them as a tea, it is wise to vary them and sometimes blend them, and not eat or drink only *one* herb many times a day, every day for months, unless prescribed by a professional. There are very reputable herbal remedy companies that make tablets and medicines, teas and ointments, which have given countless numbers of people relief from distressing illnesses.

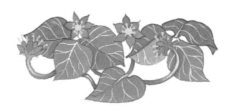

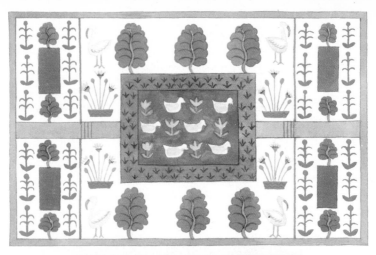

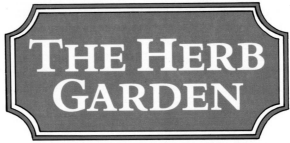

THE HERB GARDEN

The History of Herb Gardens

When human beings lived a nomadic existence in an uncivilised state, it was necessary to collect wild plants, berries and roots for food. When they became ill, instinct led them to the grasses and leaves that had curative properties, in the same way as animals do. When people began to stay in one place long enough to make a dwelling, a garden, however small, became an essential part of life. The tilling of soil and planting of herbs, vegetables and fruit trees on a plot of ground for easier gathering was a natural outcome. Plants grown for pleasure and beauty became a luxury for the aesthetic senses: special herbs and shrubs were needed for the culinary and healing properties of their foliage, flowers, or fruit, or in the stems and sometimes the roots, and often in the bark. Fragrant flowers and leaves, which were filled with perfumed essences, were made into useful and charming articles.

In ancient Egypt, excavations have uncovered perfect pictures of gardens, complete with graceful birds and brilliant butterflies, reproduced on floor tiles. Egyptian water gardens in their scale, magnitude and beauty are said to have been as breathtaking as the gardens of Versailles, constructed thousands of years later. A coloured plan on a splendid manuscript of a formal garden for an Egyptian high official in about 1390 B.C., with geometric beds intersected by paths, is still in existence and is reprinted in *Gardens in Time* by John and Ray Oldham, published by Lansdowne Press. Fruit-bearing and other trees and shrubs, waterbirds on ponds, a tangle of grape vines, pavilions, sculpted-looking plants (which may be herbs), are all depicted in a pleasing, perfect pattern and scale. There is also an illustration of an impression of the wondrous, many-terraced Hanging Gardens of Babylon, one of the seven wonders of the ancient world. Photographed pictures of superb formal gardens of early Persia, ancient Greece and the Roman and Byzantine empires show how old is the urge to make gardens of beauty, and of self-sufficiency. Indian gardens were built long before the birth of Christ. Pleasure gardens planted with flowers and trees were made more beautiful by the presence of peacocks and song birds; there were lakes for fish, the surface starred with lotus blossoms and water lilies where swans and ducks swam. These legendary Indian gardens, some intricately designed with "water ladders" and sparkling water jets, are still to be seen in Kashmir.

Old documents illustrate delightful formal gardens of the well-to-do in mediaeval Europe and in English Tudor gardens. They show how strongly dominant the impact was of early Eastern garden designs. The formality of plant beds divided into precise shapes in monastery cloisters, and in Elizabethan herb gardens and pleasure gardens, owe the origins of their plans to this Eastern influence.

Simple cottage gardens in Europe and England, and later in America and Australia, possessed their own charm with more random planting, and herbs were placed where they would be within easy reach, or if there were hives, perfumed herbs were close by, for bees love the sweet nectar of thyme, lemon balm, rosemary, sage, marjoram, oregano, borage and many more. Honey flavoured with herbs has the most delicate aroma and taste.

Suggestions for Making a Herb Garden

A simple, neat herb garden is one that is about four metres square, well-drained, and situated in a sunny position. The bed should be prepared by digging in plenty of leaf mould and mushroom or household compost. Add a small amount of coarse river sand if the soil is heavy.

If on the other hand the soil is sandy, and herbs like to grow in this type of soil for drainage, it may be built up with compost for nourishment. Beach sand is not suitable as it contains too much salt, which will kill the plants; river sand bought commercially contains no salt.

Herbs make excellent rockery plants. We once planned a rockery herb garden for friends. It was on sloping ground and herbs were planted on terraces where pathways on each level led down by steps to the small, grassy lawn below.

There are more elaborate herb gardens that one can make, such as modified mediaeval cloister gardens, and

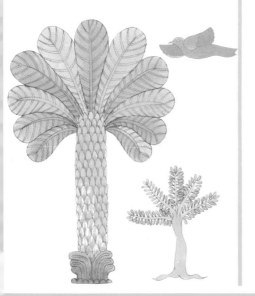

Tudor and Elizabethan gardens reminiscent of the formal ancient Eastern gardens. "Knot" gardens became popular in Tudor times and they were delineated by clipped, dwarf box hedges in complicated patterns. Fragrant, culinary, and medicinal herbs and favourite flowers were planted within the knot's miniature hedges. Scented lavender or rosemary are excellent for surrounding a garden and may be shaped and pruned after flowering. These kinds of gardens are interesting to plant and are relatively inexpensive to make.

Stone or brick walls around a herb garden cost more, but they give a special, nostalgic feeling of bygone days as you enter them. A sunken garden can be included in a more elaborate herb garden. The sides hold back the earth with paving stones, and between them, in spaces allowed for this, are planted various ornamental perfumed thymes, prostrate rosemary and small, sprawling, old-fashioned perennials, which all help to bind the soil. Low-growing herbs are planted along stone or brick pathways bisecting conventional geometric beds filled with taller herbs.

However small, a herb garden is a unique place with a definite feeling of mystique. It needs an interesting focal point like a sundial, a suitable statue, a bird-bath, or a "herb seat". This is made of brick or stone, filled with earth and covered with a matting, scented thyme or starry-flowered lawn chamomile. Paths of mown grass, paving stones, pebbles or pine bark make for easier access when picking. Small plants for edging are chives, chervil, lemon thyme, savory, upland cress, bush basil and curled parsley. Behind them, for graduated height, can be grown borage, lemon balm, sweet basil, bergamot, marjoram, French sorrel, oregano, Florence fennel, tarragon, coriander and dill. Some taller herbs for background planting are angelica, lovage, garlic, upright rosemary, Italian parsley and chicory. Bay trees grow very big if allowed to, and they can be planted on each side of the entrance to the garden; they can always be clipped and shaped to keep them compact. Elder trees and lemon verbena trees may be placed as sheltering and protective guardians just outside the herb garden.

Another way to make a pretty and pleasant herb garden is to buy an old cart wheel. Remove every second spoke and paint it white. Lay it on prepared ground and plant herbs between the spokes radiating from the centre, choosing low-growing herbs that will not sprawl all over the wheel. A similar idea is to use an old ladder, cut in half, painted white, and laid on the ground with a pathway along the centre. Herbs can be planted between the rungs.

If a herb garden as such is not important to you, and yet you would like to have a few of your favourites, grow them amongst other plants. Gardens edged with curled parsley, or chives, are useful and attractive at the same time. Taller herbs amongst other flowers add their share of fragrance and foliage interest. The larger herbs can be grown amongst the shrubs at the back of the garden.

Ingenuity plays a large part in making a herb garden, and imagination can produce some wonderful new ideas. A garden of herbs is extremely useful in many ways, as well as being full of fragrance and delicious flavours, and is always a pleasure to look at. It is worth remembering not to overfeed herbs, this makes them soft and lush with little flavour. (Parsley and chives are exceptions.) Overwatering, or a place which becomes waterlogged in heavy rain, is disastrous, although watercress is one herb that likes these conditions.

A flower garden in Shakespeare's time

"The wholesome sage, and lavender still gray
Ranke smelling rue, and cummin good for eyes
The roses, reigning in the pride of May
Sharp hishop, good for greens woundes remedies.
Fair marigolds, and bees alluring thyme,
Sweet marjoram, and daysies in their prime,
Cool violets, and Alpine growing still,
Embalmed balm, and cheerful galingale,
Dull popie, and drink quickning setual,
Veyne-healing verven, and head purging dill
Sound savorie, and basil harti-hale,
Fat coleworts, and comforting parsline,
Colde lettuce, and refreshing rosemarie,
And whatso else of vertue, good or ill,
Grew in this garden, fetched from far away
Of everyone, he takes and tastes at will."

from "The Fate of the Butterfly" by Edmund Spenser

A Shakespeare Garden

Shakespeare had a countryman's joy and delight in the herbs and flowers of hedgerows, meadows and gardens, with which he was so familiar during his rural upbringing. He loved them for the sake of their beauty, meaning and perfume, and wove many of them into his plays and sonnets.

We made a Shakespeare garden some years ago and beside each herb and flower a small notice was inscribed with the appropriate quotation on it. The size and shape of the Shakespeare plot may follow any of the suggestions for herb gardens already described but the special atmosphere that is evoked in a Shakespeare garden needs a few of Shakespeare's own words to complete the magic.

Our Shakespeare garden is oblong with a paved area in front of it and a garden seat nearby so that one can relax and contemplate at leisure. A clipped, dwarf box hedge gives it a slightly formal air and a statue of a small boy placed under a curved bower of miniature climbing roses is the focal point. In the foreground are low-growing matting thymes:

"I know a bank whereon the wild thyme blows."

A Midsummer Night's Dream

Clustered in several places are golden clumps of cowslips, oxlips and primroses.

"The even mead that erst brought sweetly forth
The freckled cowslip, burnet and sweet clover."

Henry V

And "bold" oxlips, which seem to look halfway between a cowslip and a primrose:

> "... Bold oxlips and
> The crown imperial."
>
> *The Winter's Tale*

He describes primroses many times, especially noting their ethereal beauty:

> "Pale primroses
> That die unmarried ere they can behold
> Bold Phoebus in his strength."
>
> *The Winter's Tale*

Pretty *Bellis perennis*, or pink and white English daisies, are grouped together in a rosy glow:

> "When daisies pied and violets blue,
>   And lady-smocks all silver-white,
> and cuckoo-buds of yellow hue
>   Do paint the meadows with delight."
>
> *Love's Labour's Lost*

Columbines are planted in front of the box hedge and their old-fashioned bluebonnet flowers nod above their delicate foliage:

> "There's fennel for you and columbines."
>
> *Hamlet*

Grey-leaved carnations and "gilly-vors" (a smaller type of carnation) are in this collection near the columbines, their flowering time sometimes coinciding – according to the season:

> "... the fairest flowers o' the season
> Are our carnations, and streak'd
> gillyvors."
>
> *The Winter's Tale*

The early form of pansy, before it became a giant hybrid, was *Viola tricolour,* and thank goodness it is still with us, and goes by many names – heartsease, love-in-idleness, Johnny-jump-up, and cupid's flower are a few. The plant is massed with tiny pansy-like flowers of purple and gold in spring; it self-sows readily and since it is an annual its little pod of seeds, which ripen after flowering, burst open and fall on the ground, the welcome seedlings appearing again year after year. We let it grow unchecked, and remember that it was the flower Oberon told Puck to find to put Titania to sleep in *A Midsummer Night's Dream:*

> ... And maidens call it Love-in-idleness.
> Fetch me that flower: the herb I show'd
>   thee once;
> The juice of it, on sleeping eyelids laid,
> Will make or man or woman madly dote
> Upon the next live creature that it sees."

A silver-grey wormwood hedge surrounds the garden, and appropriately it was the herb Oberon used to awaken Titania, and called more delightfully by Shakespeare "Dian's bud":

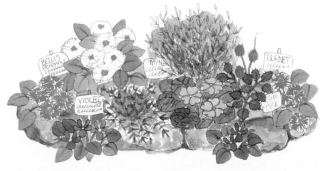

"Be, as thou was wont to be:
See as thou was wont to see;
Dian's bud o'er Cupid's flower
Hath such force and blessed power.
Now, my Titania! wake you, my sweet
   queen."
                A Midsummer Night's Dream.

There are many more herbs and flowers to plant in a Shakespeare garden. The white Florentine iris, *Iris germanica,* or "Fair Flower-de-Luce".
                                    Henry V.

All the herbs mentioned in these lines from *The Winter's Tale* are in the garden:

"Hot lavender", mints, savory and marjoram.

There is a rosemary bush for Ophelia:

"There's rosemary, that's for remembrance; pray you love, remember."
                                    Hamlet

and also rue, the "Herb of Grace":

"There's rue for you;
And here's some for me;
We may call it herb-grace o' Sundays:
O you must wear your rue with a
   difference."
                                    Hamlet

Honeysuckle, the early form with small, scented creamy flowers, and often called "woodbine", is a reminder of Titania's bower "over-canopied with lush woodbine" in *A Midsummer Night's Dream.*

There must be roses in a Shakespeare garden. As well as the rose arch which enshrines the small statue in our garden, there are other historic old roses planted outside its confines to catch the sun and air: they include the white rose of York and the red rose of Lancaster, which historically eventually became united in the red and white Tudor rose:

"We will unite the white rose and the red.
Smile, heaven upon this fair conjunction."
                                    Richard III.

The cuckoo-bud or buttercup we did not plant because of its invasive root system, nor do we have lady-smocks, harebells or eglantine, simply because there is no more room! Daffodils are in other parts of the garden, as are violets, fennel and marigolds.

There is a crabapple tree in one corner of the Shakespeare garden. A favourite drink in The Bard's day was roasted crabapples dropped into ale:

"When roasted crabs hiss in the bowl
Then nightly sings the staring owl."
                                    Love's Labour's Lost

Hemlock, fennel and crowflower, or ragged robin, are a few more of the many other "Shakespeare" plants.

Bible Gardens

We have always intended to create a "Bible garden", especially after reading about one in an overseas magazine some time ago. Like a Shakespeare garden, the herbs, flowers and trees of a Bible garden need notices next to them with the appropriate quotations and the name of the herb clearly written on them.

A garden such as this need not be large, although the design would be important – a simple square with a suitable central focus, such as a bird-bath or a small statue, would suffice. Paths could radiate outwards from the centre, and plants set in beds bordering the paths.

Some of the herbs quoted in the Bible are the bitter herbs such as dandelion, chicory and sorrel. Bitter herbs have a symbolic use in the Jewish annual Passover ceremony. Fennel, cumin and rue are some of the other herbs referred to in the Bible. Wormwood is mentioned in Amos 5:7:

"Ye who turn judgment to wormwood, and leave off righteousness in the earth."

Aromatic coriander seed appears in Exodus 16:31:

"And the house of Israel called the name thereof Manna: and it *was* like coriander seed, white; and the taste of it *was* like wafers *made* with honey."

Leeks, onions and garlic, all members of the Allium family, appear in Numbers 11:5:

"We remember the fish, which we did eat in Egypt freely; the cucumbers, and the melons, and the leeks, and the onions, and the garlick."

Other plants that could be put in or around a Bible garden, and which are all named, are broom, lilies, the cedar of Lebanon, grapevines, fruit trees, and in the right areas, date palms, sycamores, and of course, spices:

"Spikenard and saffron; calamus and cinnamon, with all trees of frankincense; myrrh and aloes, with all the chief spices." (Song of Solomon 4:15)

It would of course be difficult or even impossible to include the larger species, and tropical plants bearing spices, because of lack of space or unsuitability of the climate, but creating a garden with a meaning and a story behind it would give pleasure and satisfaction to both the beholder and the creator of the garden.

It was a wonderful experience to see the re-creation of a true 17th century Culpeper garden at romantic Leed's Castle in Kent, on a perfect summer's day. We wandered through paths set between beds of herbs, both culinary and medicinal, as well as flowers, surrounded by low hedges trimmed in different patterns. We were grateful to the person who had so faithfully re-created this garden that it looked exactly as it would have in Culpeper's day.

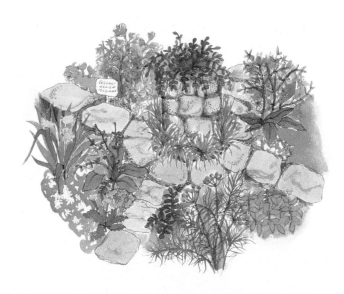

Propagating herbs

There are many people who are keen cooks and who would like to use fresh herbs from their gardens or be able to make herb teas and simple remedies, potpourris and pomanders. But they may not feel they are competent gardeners – "I haven't got green fingers, only a purple thumb," they say! For those people the solution would be to buy established plants from a nursery and then put them in a sunny position in the garden, within easy reach of the kitchen.

A herb garden requires a patch of well-forked soil about four metres square. There are three ways to propagate herb plants – by seed, cuttings, or by root division.

Sowing seed

Herbs are sown in spring. In climates where winters are mild, some may be sown again in the autumn. Seeds of most annuals can be sown directly into their permanent position in a prepared bed. Perennials, being much slower growers, fare better if seeds are sown into containers filled with a fine potting mixture where they can be more easily cared for until they are 2 or 3 cm high and have begun to take root. The seedlings should then be carefully removed from the pot and planted in the garden, making sure that the soil does not fall away from the roots in the process.

When filling a seed tray or pot, use a fine, light mixture of soil. An excellent combination is made up of two parts of sandy loam to one part of coarse river sand, one part of peat moss and, for nourishment, 1 gm of blood and bone to 1 litre of soil mixture. Alternatively, a fine soil can be bought in bags from your local nursery and is called "potting mix".

When putting it into a seed-box or pots, make sure it is 0.5 cm below the edge of the container to allow for watering. Commercial packs of seed-starting trays or pots, comprising specially prepared compressed peat moss, are available from most nurseries, and this is an even simpler way of raising herbs from seeds. Instructions are given on the packs.

When sowing seeds straight into the ground, water the bed well beforehand, then scatter seeds, or sow in drills, and cover with fine soil (rubbed between the hands) to approximately twice the thickness of the seed. Press down lightly on the earth with a flat piece of wood to pack it tightly around the seeds. Keep moist with a light, misty spray of water until germination, when a green haze of new shoots will push their way through the surface. If seeds are allowed to dry out during germination the growing process will cease, and if this happens, no amount of watering will rejuvenate them.

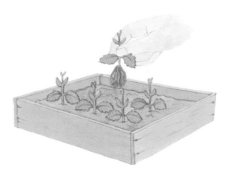

Taking Cuttings

Plants that must be grown from cuttings are a little more difficult to propagate, and judgement is needed as to which time of the season is best. This can vary from one year to the next, according to the weather. The best time to take most cuttings is in late spring after the earlier growth has hardened the new shoots. If the cutting is too soft it will wilt when put into sand. One way to determine if a cutting is hard enough is to bend it to about 70 degrees and if it springs back to its original position it is firm enough to use.

When taking cuttings in late spring use the tips of the shoots, taking 6–8 cm early in the morning before the sun has had time to wilt them, or collect what you will need on a dull day. Strip off the lower leaves, keeping two to four at the top. Always remove the foliage with an upward pull: if tugged downwards the bark will sometimes come away with the leaf, making the cutting useless. With very soft shoots, it is better to remove leaves with a sharp knife or secateurs. Trim with secateurs just below a node and make sure it is a clean cut with no jagged edges. The cutting when trimmed should be 4–6 cm long. When the cuttings have been prepared, fill a container with a mixture of coarse river sand and peat moss. A 12.5 cm pot will hold about twenty cuttings.

Before putting in the prepared shoots, dip each one in a reliable fresh cutting powder, available from nurseries. There are several strengths on the market. No. 1 is for softwood, No. 2 for semi-hardwood, and No. 3 for hardwood. One that gives good results and which saves much trouble and expense is an all-purpose cutting powder.

To push cuttings into sand, use a dibbler or a pencil to make a hole, then press the sand firmly around the stem with your finger, or the other end of the dibbler. If the cuttings are pushed into coarse sand without first making a hole, the bark might be damaged. Put the prepared filled pot of cuttings in a warm, shady place until the shoots have made roots, then plant them into individual pots containing a reliable potting mixture. Keep them well watered. If roots are showing around the soil when the plants are knocked out of the pot, they are ready to go into the herb garden.

Root division

Growing herbs by root division is the easiest way to propagate, provided you have a large stock plant that can be spared to do this. The mints are usually increased from root division, as some varieties send out runners which make roots at each leaf node. When dividing a plant, make sure that every piece you take has some rootlets attached to it. When the clump has been separated into a number of suitable pieces, put them into containers with potting soil, and keep one to use as an extra stock plant that can be divided next year.

If you are interested, and have the time to propagate your own herbs, it can become an absorbing and relaxing hobby and you will suddenly find that you have far more plants than are needed for the garden. It should not be too difficult to sell the surplus stock to nearby nurseries, provided the plants are healthy and have been grown in a conventional plastic pot. No matter how good a plant looks, a potential customer will not buy it if it is growing in a jam tin, or a yoghurt or ice-cream carton! Herbs are also extremely popular on garden stalls at fêtes. Presentation is important here too and a fair price may be charged for them if

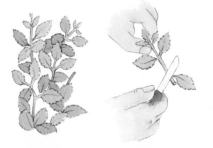

they look professional. A gift of a herb plant to friends and family is always welcome.

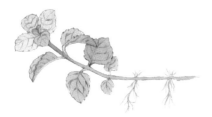

Companion planting

Plants and trees, whatever their size, are all individual, each one being a composition of many complex parts, besides the roots, trunk, stems, leaves, flowers, bark or fruit that are visible to the naked eye. Within the make-up of the plant or tree are fine substances that are either alien to other plants, trees and countless insects, or they are sympathetic to them and assist their growth and attract desirable insects to them. Companion planting is the science of finding out which plants are compatible to one another so as to eliminate the use of chemical sprays.

Root excretions and the micro-life of the soil are all-important factors and the subject is a very intricate one. There are books that deal exclusively and in depth with companion planting but we will include here a few of the facts and findings for those who would like to know something about this fascinating aspect of gardening and farming.

The impact of companion planting is not immediate, as with contact or systematic sprays. Sometimes one has to wait for a year or two before the results are manifested. For instance, if a fruit tree is susceptible to a specific disease, and a plant known to be particularly resistant to it is planted underneath, in time the fruit tree will absorb some of the root excretions and other benefits from the plant. The tree will then become unattractive to its enemy. In the same way it has been found that the roots of the French marigold (*Tagetes patula*) give off a substance which kills soil nematode worms in rose beds, the nematodes being especially harmful to the health of roses. Rachel Carson wrote of this in *Silent Spring*.

In their book *"Companion Plants"*, Helen Philbrick and Richard B. Gregg (Stuart and Watkins, London) tell us that not only the French marigold, but the African marigold too has the same properties to combat other soil nematodes, including potato nematodes. When marigolds are planted in a tomato bed, they combat white fly and the tomato plants grow better and bear more fruit. Even the odour of marigold foliage and blossoms is effective as an insect repellent.

We have found that a strong wormwood tea poured around the haunts of snails and slugs is an effective repellent. Another remarkable insect repellent is pennyroyal. Sprigs of it under a dog's mat will combat fleas, and during a flea plague sprigs of pennyroyal liberally spread around the house will get rid of the fleas. Pennyroyal growing in the garden repels mosquitoes and ants.

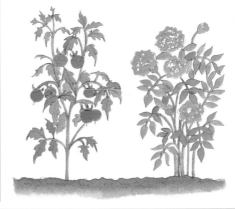

Planting Herb Gardens in Containers

Many people living in units have little or no garden in which to grow their favourite plants, much as they would like to.

Herbs are easily grown in containers, provided they have plenty of sun and air, such as on a balcony or a window sill. Herbs should never be treated as indoor plants otherwise they will become disappointingly leggy and yellow, then die.

There are many types of suitable pots to buy for container growing: popular and easily obtainable are strawberry jars which are made in various sizes. They are mainly of terracotta and are sometimes glazed on the outside in attractive colours. Terracotta containers always need to be placed on a saucer because the pots are porous, and during dry, hot weather the saucer should be filled with water so that the pot draws up moisture which keeps the plants alive.

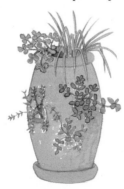

An average size strawberry jar has five or six lipped holes in the sides and one large aperture in the top. This would be suitable for a balcony. Troughs are also favourite containers for herb gardens and are made in various sizes out of many different materials, such as terracotta (some with pleasing neo-classic designs on them), cement, crushed marble and polystyrene. A fairly small trough would be practical for a kitchen window sill, the size depending on the depth of the sill.

Other types of containers that may be used for raising herbs are large, round tubs made of cement, terracotta, or old wooden wine casks cut in half. We were once offered a large, ancient Roman sink which would have looked superb planted with herbs, but unfortunately it was much too expensive!

Excellent and unusual alternatives are wire baskets lined with damp paper bark (wetting makes it pliable), which when filled can be hung from an overhead beam on a terrace or a balcony. There are also terracotta hanging pots, some with holes in the side. The attractive wicker lobster pots have become much sought after as planters: they vary in shape and size and have suitably heavy chains for hanging. Line these with damp newspaper before filling with soil and herbs. The paper eventually rots into a firm compost while preventing the soil from falling through the cane.

Yet another alternative for growing herbs in a confined area is a novel attachment for a window, which resembles a miniature glasshouse.

When looking for a suitable container for your herb garden, make sure that it has a hole, or holes, in the bottom for drainage; if the hole or holes look rather large, as they sometimes are, cover each with a rough, unevenly shaped stone. This will stop the soil in the pot from falling out and at the same time will allow any excess water to gradually drain away. Do not use a flat stone that will completely cover the hole, seal in the water and kill the plant in the waterlogged soil.

When planting out herbs from their growing pots, knock them out gently, first making sure that the soil is moist so that it does not fall away from the

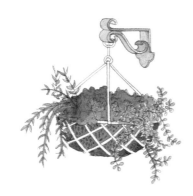

through the porous soil and repeat this about three times. By doing this you will ensure that the lowest plants in the side will get sufficient moisture.

Much as we all like to grow mint, this herb, with its invasive root system, is better off in its own pot otherwise before long it will take over the whole container and strangle all the herbs in it.

roots. Small-growing culinary herbs with compact root systems, such as thyme, chives, marjoram, sage, oregano, parsley and chervil, can be planted fairly close together and still flourish. A trough approximately 60 cm long and 20 cm wide will comfortably hold five herbs, especially if they are staggered when arranging them. A shallow azalea pot 40 cm in diameter holds up to seven plants.

Planting a strawberry jar with herbs is really quite easy once you know how. Whichever size you choose, start by putting a fairly large, uneven stone on top of the hole in the bottom and then fill the jar with potting mix to the level of the lowest lipped holes. Knock a plant from its pot and pass it down through the large opening at the top, pushing the foliage part of the herb through one of the side holes and leaving the roots intact within the pot. When all the side apertures are planted at this level, fill the pot with more soil to the next level of apertures and repeat the same process as before. When the top has been reached, plant with one of the larger herbs, like rosemary, leaving 2 cm from the top for watering. Never fill a strawberry jar with soil and sow seeds in the lipped holes because they will wash out when watering.

To water a strawberry or herb jar, fill the pot to the very top, let it soak

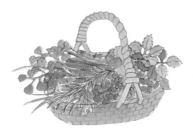

Harvesting and drying herbs

When drying herbs it is important that the watery element should evaporate, leaving behind the fragrant essential oils which contain many other components as well. The reason that dried herbs have a stronger taste than fresh herbs is because the oils are concentrated in the shrunken, demoisturised leaves. In cooking, if you are using dried herbs instead of fresh herbs, use only half the amount suggested in the recipe.

There are several ways of drying your own herbs. If you are drying them for their aromatic foliage, a general rule is to gather them on a dry day, before noon, when they are at their peak. After that, the sun will have drawn up most of the aromatic essences. Early autumn, just before flowering, is the usual time for harvesting. Oregano is the exception. An Italian friend told us that, in his Sicilian homeland, oregano is harvested and dried when it is in flower. The most intense flavour is in the flower heads, and these are used as well as the leaves for their extreme pungency. (Never hesitate to eat culinary herb flowers, fresh or dried, as well as the leaves: thyme, marjoram and savory are three that come to mind – their flavour is lightly honeyed as well as aromatic, and they harmonise perfectly with their foliage.) When harvesting herbs, cut each plant off at ground level, and if they are perennials they will appreciate the pruning.

The simplest way to dry herbs is to bundle them together neatly in bunches, tie with string or raffia, and hang them in an airy, shady, dust-free place until brittle. Then strip off the leaves and put them into clean, airtight containers; do not use plastic, it causes "sweating". We used to recommend that herbs be washed first, but on reading one knowledgeable writer's comment that some of the natural essences clinging to the plant would be lost, we no longer advocate this, unless of course the herbs have been sprayed with insecticide. There is also a chance of mildew setting in if the foliage is damp.

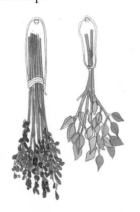

For really efficient, natural drying, branchlets of herbs can be laid on airy, mesh trays in a warm, dry atmosphere where the air can circulate around them. Spreading the herbs on sheets of clean newspaper and leaving them in a shady area is also an excellent method. If the leaves are the type that retain moisture, to prevent mould or mildew from forming, place them so that they do not have any contact with each other. Never dry foliage in the sun, it will draw out all the flavour, neither should they be dried in a *hot* oven. A warm oven is satisfactory provided the leafy stalks are constantly turned and carefully watched. Drying in a microwave oven can be successful and this method is described below.

If the heads of herbs are to be dried for the seed, as in the Umbelliferae family, which includes fennel and dill, then final sun-drying is excellent.

Washed sprays of fresh herbs, as well as chopped fresh herbs, can be wrapped in foil or plastic film and stored in the refrigerator for a week. They may also be deep-frozen for up to three weeks. To keep them fresh for longer, wash the herbs, chop finely and freeze in ice cube trays with a little water. When needed, defrost the frozen herbs, or drop the ice cubes into the cooking pot where the ice will soon melt. Herb butters are another way to keep your herbs fresh. Most culinary herbs are suitable for herb butters. Wash each batch and chop finely before incorporating into softened butter, with a few drops of lemon juice added. Spread the herb butter onto a fairly deep saucer or plate, and refrigerate. When hard, cut into circles or cubes, put them into a covered container, or a plastic bag, secure the top and freeze until needed.

Basil is the least satisfactory herb to freeze, it is inclined to discolour and become bitter. As mentioned in *Herbs, Their Cultivation and Usage* (page 99) ,

Mrs Clare Wilmot's easy recipe for Pestou, a superb thick basil sauce, is the most delicious way of preserving fresh basil.

Herb vinegars, for use in French dressings, are a pleasant way of capturing summer flavours. These are described on page 104.

Drying Herbs in a Microwave Oven

We sought the advice of an expert on microwave cookery who considers microwave drying a very efficient and quick method of drying herbs. It is advisable to first do a few trial runs, leaving the herbs that have been microwave dried for two or three weeks in airtight containers to establish that they have dried and not developed mould. For future refer-ence, it is important to make a note of how long each herb was in the oven.

After picking the herbs, wash and pat dry with a paper towel. Turn the oven on to full power and lay whole herb sprays, or stripped, fresh foliage, on two layers of absorbent paper on an ovenproof dish. The paper helps to absorb excess moisture. Most herbs seem to dry in about four minutes. Feel them, and if they are not crisp, leave them a little longer, making sure they do not discolour. Each herb varies in drying time, so even half a minute could be crucial. Chervil takes as little as one minute to dry, and chives a little more than four minutes. Parsley is particularly rewarding, becoming an even brighter green then when picked from the garden. Dried, whole sprigs look very attractive.

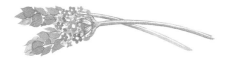

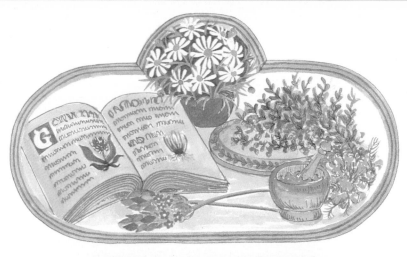

ALL ABOUT HERBS

We are continually in contact with thousands of people and it is always gratifying to recognise the keen interest in herbs that is shown by men, women, and even teenagers. Everybody wants to know more and more about herbs, which bears out our theory that this quest for knowledge is an inherited folk memory that most of us seem to carry unconsciously within ourselves, and which many cultures in other countries, particularly in Asia, have never lost.

It would take volumes to analyse and describe every wild or cultivated herb, so in this book we have chosen to write about a general range of herbs which are easily found in specialist herb nurseries, either as seedlings or as seeds. They all have culinary, nutritional, and healing uses; some have cosmetic value as well, and all these attributes are discussed in detail.

The famous astrologer-physician, Dr Nicholas Culpeper, who lived in the seventeenth century and whose works are still being published, made some delightful and helpful astrological observations on herbs, and in this book we have quoted many of these.

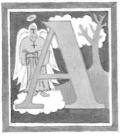

ANGELICA

(*Angelica archangelica*) Umbelliferae
Biennial

Angelica has been described as one of the "stately" herbs. It grows to 1.5–2 m (5–8 ft) and is one of the tallest herbs not classified as a shrub or a small tree. The whole plant exudes a fine, sweetish fragrance but it is more pronounced in the hollow, bronze-green stems and stalks. The large, round, creamy-lime flower heads bloom in spring, usually in their second year, and the tiny flowerets, which make up the composite bloom, have a piercing, aromatic flavour. The ripened flower seeds should be collected immediately because their germinating period lasts no longer than two weeks. Sowing the seed is the usual method of propagation, or sometimes by division of old roots, or by offshoots from the main stem, but these methods are less satisfactory. If stinging nettle is grown near angelica the essential oil in angelica is increased by more than 80 per cent.

This handsome herb is a native of northern Europe and thrives in a moist, shady position.

There is another, smaller, variety of angelica which has ornamental, curled, glossy leaves (*A. pachycarpa*). It is not as high in medicinal properties, although the flavour is good both for candying the stalks and for making a refreshing tea.

The Archangel Raphael is said to have appeared to a monk in a dream during a time of plague and revealed that a piece of stalk or root held in the mouth and chewed would drive away the dreaded peril. Because of its angelic associations it became known as "angelica". Another name for it was "the rooth of the Holy Ghost". According to the 17th century herbalist, Culpeper, it is a herb of the sun in Leo.

Uses:

Culinary – The stalks and stems are crystallised and used to decorate cakes and desserts. The fresh young leaves may be finely chopped and added to salads. They give a delicate flavour to stewed fruit and may be used in the preparation of jellies and preserves. The roots are sometimes sliced and cooked as a vegetable.

Medicinal – The whole plant possesses digestive properties and Angelica is also excellent for inducing perspiration and may be used as an expectorant. It soothes smoker's cough and is sometimes used to treat anaemia as well as being taken as a general tonic. Angelica taken as a tea is helpful as a remedy for flatulence.

In cold weather a refreshing and warming drink may be made from the leaves, although it is mainly the root which is used to make the tea which is said to have curative properties. People with a tendency to diabetes are warned against taking angelica, as it has a tendency to produce sugar in the urine.

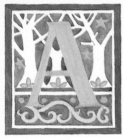

ANISE

(Pimpinella anisum) Umbelliferae
Annual

Anise is a small, parsley-like plant 45–60 cm (1½–2 ft) high with serrated leaves that have a warmly aromatic taste. The flat, white flower heads are followed by intensely fragrant fruit or seeds which ripen to a brown colour and have the typical aniseed flavour. The plant prefers a sheltered, sunny position in light, well-drained soil. Propagation is by seed in spring, and in mild climates it may be sown again in autumn. Coriander and anise plants grow well together, each improving the quality of their fruit in every way.

Anise is native to Middle Eastern countries; it was cultivated by the ancient Egyptians and Greeks and was mentioned in the Bible. During the Middle Ages it became widely known in Europe and was valued for the fruit, which has strong digestive properties. The quality of the seeds was also known by the early Romans who used them with other aromatic seeds in special fruit cakes, not only for the pleasant taste, but to help the digestion. Anise is also used to flavour soups, ground seeds being more suitable for this than whole seeds.

Aniseed is widely used in the preparation of liqueurs. In hot weather, a most refreshing drink can be made by half filling a tumbler with ice, then adding two or three teaspoons of Anisette liqueur and topping up with ice-cold water.

Star-anise (*Illicium anisatum*), a spice with a taste very similar to anise, comes from a small tree native to China. It has an attractive seed, larger than aniseed, brown, hard, and shaped like a tiny star – hence its name. It too has excellent digestive properties and is widely used for this purpose and also as a flavouring in Oriental food.

To harvest the seeds of anise, allow the flowers to set their fruit and when brownish in colour, cut off the heads before the seeds drop. Store them in cardboard boxes and expose them to direct sunlight occasionally to completely dry them out. When crisp and dry, shake the flower heads so that most of the seeds fall out, then sift them through a sieve, removing any remaining husks and bits of flower heads. Store the seeds in clean, airtight jars.

Uses:

Culinary – Whole or ground aniseed gives food a delicious flavour and makes it easier to digest. Aniseed is used in many types of bread, cakes and biscuits and may be used to add a delicious flavour to cooked, buttered carrots, turnips and beetroot. Cook some of the whole seed when steaming cabbage, and sprinkle it into coleslaw. When baking apples or pears, shake a few seeds on to the fruit while cooking. Aniseed may be used instead of caraway seed, which has similar digestive properties and is not unlike it in flavour. Put a few of the fresh leaves in a green salad.

Medicinal – Aniseed is said to have many beneficial qualities. It may be used to relieve certain respiratory disorders as well as indigestion and flatulence. It is also helpful in alleviating colds and influenza, and is said to strengthen and brighten the eyes. Aniseed tea is refreshing to the palate and sweetens the breath. Anise is used to flavour cough lozenges, some cordials and tea blends. A *very weak* aniseed tea is a helpful beverage for soothing children, especially if they have colic; it should be mixed with warm milk and a little honey. It is interesting to note that Anisette liqueur is said to be helpful in cases of bronchitis and is considered to have a favourable effect on the bronchial tubes.

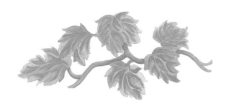

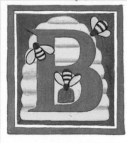

BALM

(Melissa officinalis) Labiatae
Perennial

This refreshingly lemon-scented herb is propagated by seeds, cuttings, and root division in spring, and in temperate climates again in autumn. It likes moist, rich soil and sunshine for part of the day. It grows to 75 cm (2½ ft) or more, depending on soil and rainfall.

Although a member of the mint family, the shallow roots of balm (or lemon balm as it is often called) are not invasive and it can be grown in a herb garden quite easily. In summer, from being a low, leafy clump, the plant increases in height and sends out flower stalks with clusters of tiny white blooms climbing up them. Bees are very much attracted to balm blossoms (its botanic name of *Melissa* is derived from a Greek word meaning bee).

The fragrant leaves when dried are an excellent addition to a potpourri blend. Balm planted near vegetables increases their flavour and resistance to diseases.

Balm has been highly regarded amongst herbs for many centuries, and the name is derived from "balsam" which ranks high as a source of sweet-smelling oils.

This herb is native to the mountainous regions of southern Europe and has spread widely in the course of time through England, North America and parts of Asia.

Culpeper, who described all the plants he wrote about as being under the influence of specific heavenly bodies, says "It is an herb of Jupiter and under Cancer and strengthens the body in all its actions".

Uses:

Culinary — Fresh lemon balm leaves, finely chopped and mixed with half the amount of chopped chives, make a delicious seasoning for chicken, fish, lamb or pork. Balm leaves also enhance the flavour of cooked, buttered vegetables. Whole, washed balm leaves look attractive and lend their subtle fragrance to both fruit and savoury salads. For an old and tried pick-me-up, which also tastes pleasant, add a little fresh or dried balm to a pot of Indian tea.

Medicinal — The wonderful properties of balm are manifold; it eases griping pains and helps to dispel flatulence, while having a tonic effect on the stomach. Balm is also excellent for influenza as it induces mild perspiration. It aids the digestion and increases the appetite. It revives one on a hot day and is soothing as well. The early herbalists believed that it prevented senility and impotence and contributed to longevity. It was also believed to drive away melancholy, causing "the mind and heart to become merry..." Culpeper also claimed that it was good for the liver and spleen and that it eased the pain of gout.

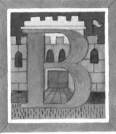

BASIL

(Ocimum basilicum) Labiatae
Annual

Basil, together with French tarragon, is one of the most highly regarded culinary herbs. It is propagated by sowing seeds in late spring or early summer. An earlier sowing will often end in disappointment, for a late cold snap will kill the tender new plants overnight. All of the many varieties prefer a sunny, sheltered position in light to sandy, well-drained soil. Sweet basil *(Ocimum basilicum)* grows to 75 cm (2½ ft) while bush basil *(O. minimum)*, which is denser and more compact in form, only reaches a height of 30 cm (12 inches). These two varieties have white flowers, which should be discouraged from blooming too soon. This is easily done by pinching out the centres of the plant which will promote bushy, branching stems and prolong the use of the leaves. If basil is allowed to go its own way, it will send up flower stems too quickly and become spindly and will not be of much use as a culinary herb.

In companion planting, basil grown with tomatoes helps to repel the dreaded white fly which attacks this vegetable. Do not plant basil near rue as they are not compatible and will inhibit each other's growth.

Both sweet and bush basil seeds and seedlings are easily obtained from most nurseries and are the most traditional for culinary purposes. There is a highly ornamental basil *(O. dark opal)* with purple-magenta foliage, and when the attractive pale pink blooms are in flower they are constantly surrounded by bees. The perfume of the leaves and flowers is very pronounced, the leaf being coarser in texture than green basil; however sprigs of this basil used as a garnish, and some whole leaves mixed into a green salad, give perfume and colour. Among some of the basils encountered lately, and which are put out by specialist seedsmen, are licorice basil, lemon basil, green bouquet basil, cinnamon basil, lettuce leaf basil, monstrous basil, piccolo basil, sacred basil, tree basil, camphor basil and perennial basil. Camphor basil is recommended as a perennial (perhaps not in areas which have extremely cold and snowy winters) and its dried leaves make an excellent moth repellent. The aroma of the foliage is not at all appetising; it smells exactly like camphor. Tree basil's leaves are bright green and coarse with a typical basil perfume; it has reddish stems and grows to approximately 1.5 m (5 ft). It is not a variety that should be used raw, but chopped finely it is excellent for dishes that require slow cooking. It can be added with other ingredients at the beginning.

Basil is surrounded by folklore that goes back thousands of years. It was known to the ancient Egyptians,

Greeks and Romans. The different types of basil seem to have originated in various countries, among them being India, Japan, Java, Malaysia, and of course the Mediterranean countries.

Culpeper says it is "A herb of Mars and under the Scorpion, and therefore called Basilicon..."

Uses:

Culinary – Wherever this delectable herb is grown it is used in countless ways in the preparation of food. It is the main ingredient in the delicious Italian sauce *pestou* and the French *soupe au pistou*. It goes well with tomatoes, either cooked or raw. The finely chopped leaves can be sprinkled over cooked, buttered vegetables and it can be added to vegetable soups during the last half hour of cooking. Mix the chopped leaves with cream cheese as a sandwich filling, or as a party dip. Left whole, the leaves enliven a mixed green salad and it is traditionally used in pasta dishes, as is oregano.

Medicinal – Basil has many therapeutic qualities. It aids the digestion and helps to expel flatulence. It has also been used as a herbal remedy for "the brain, heart and lungs", and diseases of the kidneys and bladder. It has also been used for some nervous disorders (see the chapter on Herb Teas). In India it is sacred to the gods Krishna and Vishnu, and is regarded as a herb fit for a king.

The dried, powdered leaves are made into a snuff which is used to relieve nervous headaches.

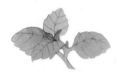

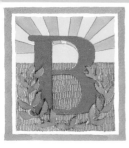

BAY TREE

(Laurus nobilis) Lauraceae
Perennial

The noble bay tree is native to the Mediterranean countries and grows to a height of at least 11 m (40 ft) in good quality soil in an open, sunny position. The pungent leaves flavour certain foods. Both leaves and berries yield an oil which has many uses in herbal medicine. Propagation is by sowing seed or by taking cuttings in spring. Cuttings are a more satisfactory way of increasing stock because the seeds do not germinate easily. In companion planting, the aromatic quality of the tree enlivens the essences of plants growing in the vicinity. The tree sends up many suckers and one would imagine that this would be a quick and easy way of propagation; however these suckers do not have roots of their own as they are joined to the parent tree and it is wise to cut them off at ground level before they become too tall.

Bay trees are sometimes affected by a disease called white wax scale which can be treated effectively in the early stages. While the tree is small, use a clean rag to rub the leaves with a mild solution of detergent and water. If the tree is too large to go over it leaf by leaf, spray it well all over and under the foliage with white oil (which is not harmful) starting in late spring when the pest which causes the scale begins to be active, and continue this treatment methodically once a month until late summer.

The tree blooms in mid to late spring, and bees love the intensely scented, nectar-filled puffballs of golden flowers.

There are abundant historical associations connected with the bay laurel. In ancient Greece and Rome the leaves were fashioned into chaplets to honour outstanding sportsmen, men of letters, and the bravest of soldiers. The tradition is carried on to this day in that the leaves are incorporated into the design of Royal Air Force badges... little do we realise how ancient and significant are many of today's symbols!

In Culpeper's astrology concerning the bay he says: "It is a tree of the Sun and under the celestial sign of Leo, and resisteth witchcraft very patently, as also all the evils old Saturn can do the body of man, and they are not a few".

Uses:

Culinary – Bay leaves are widely used in cooking and comprise part of a "bouquet garni" or posy of savoury herbs which include parsley, marjoram and thyme; sometimes a few peppercorns and a stalk of celery are added. These are all tied together so that they can be removed later. A bouquet garni may also be dried first, crushed finely and put into small muslin bags so that the flavour is imparted during long, slow cooking and then the bag is removed at the last minute.

A dried, crushed bouquet garni is also available loose, and long cooking softens all the herbs which amalagamate into the juices of the dish. Fresh or dried whole bay leaves may be used on their own during baking or steaming, and also flavour sauces, marinades and terrines.

Medicinal – The leaves and berries yield a volatile oil by distillation. When prescribed by a qualified herbalist, the oil has properties which are beneficial for treating rheumatic complaints, hysteria, flatulence, and as an aid to digestion. It was said that the oil relieved earache when administered in drops. A beneficial weak tea may be made with the fresh or dried leaves. Externally, oil of bay is used to ease the pain of sprains and bruises. One writer with insight into the more ethereal benefits of herbs says that the functions of the sweet bay laurel are directed to the head and nerves and to the consciousness, and that through the process of nutrition, symbolically crown the head with the forces of light.

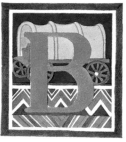

BERGAMOT

(Monarda didyma) Labiatae
Perennial

This native of North America is one of the most sweetly fragrant herbs. It has mint-like foliage and honeyed heads of tousled blossoms. Propagation is by seed or root division, and sometimes cuttings, in spring. The best position for the plant is where the roots will be cool in summer, and where the 1.20 m (4 ft) stems can catch the sun. It is ideally placed behind other shorter herbs which will shade the roots, and where the lovely blooms can be seen. It likes rich, moist soil, and if it is growing near other plants that dislike these conditions, a light dressing of old, powdery poultry manure or compost may be spread over the base of the plant and a fine sprinkler directed to the lower part of the herb in hot, dry weather.

Flowers of bergamot may vary from white, shell-pink and different shades of mauve to bright crimson. The hardiest of all is the latter, "Cambridge Scarlet'. In spring the stems begin to rise from the leaf-matted base, and blooming begins in summer. Each flower head is a mass of long, tubular petals overflowing with nectar. Pick one or two when passing and enjoy the subtle, fragrant "drink of the gods", but leave plenty for the honey-eating birds in the garden and for the bees, who adore it: one of its old names was "bee balm". Another name for bergamot was "Oswego

Tea" because an infusion of the leaves was widely used by the Oswego Indians and this beverage soon became popular with the new settlers from the Old World.

A Spanish physician, Nicholas Monardes, discovered the herb in the 16th century, which is why it has the botanical name of *Monarda*. The dried leaves and flowers are an excellent addition to a potpourri.

Uses:

Culinary – The young leaves and torn-up flowers give a delicious flavour to a green salad. It can be used instead of sage in veal dishes; it also combines well with pork. Chop the leaves finely and sprinkle them over cooked, buttered vegetables. Whole young leaves impart their delicate aroma to a fruit salad. A leafy stalk plunged into long glasses of icy cold drinks, or into a jug of fruit juice, gives a delectable, elusive fragrance.

Medicinal – A tea made with the fresh or dried leaves is said to be beneficial for fevers or an upset stomach and has even been found to be soothing to the nerves. The American Indians used the tea for colds, sore throats and bronchial ailments. Being a member of the mint family, it has been found to contain an antiseptic oil called thymol.

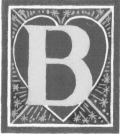

BORAGE

(Borago officinalis) Boraginaceae
Annual

Although borage is an annual, it self-sows prolifically and often its grey-green foliage and modestly bowed heads of sky-blue flowers and fat buds, softly misted with downy calyxes, appear in unexpected corners of the garden. We let it grow in unusual places because somehow it always seems to be the most harmonious filling for patches of garden that could have been uninteresting. Now and again one pink blossom will appear among the blue. Propagation is by seed all through the year in mild climates. Where winters are exceptionally cold, seed is sown in spring. The best position for the plant is in a sheltered place in semi-shade, and this is the sort of spot where it self-sows and reaches grand proportions. Its usual height is 90 cm (3 ft) but it can grow taller. The stems are thick and rather soft and are covered with bristly hairs, as are the leaves, especially the lower, larger ones. Both foliage and flowers have uses in cooking and medicine.

Aleppo is said to be the original home of borage. It has spread widely in every country where it has been introduced, and even grows in poor ground; however, the better the soil, the more the plant will flourish. Bees are attracted to the nectar-filled blossoms, and honey from borage flowers

is particularly delectable. In companion planting, borage and strawberries are compatible, the borage usually being planted on the edges of the beds because when it grows very tall some branches will begin to hang down and smother nearby plants.

In astrology it is under the signs of Jupiter and Leo – "great strengtheners of nature"

Uses:

Culinary – Borage stems and leaves are high in saline mucilage, as well as containing potassium, calcium and mineral acids. When dried it contains a certain percentage of potash and when burnt the presence of the latter will send forth sparks. In France the flowers are widely used to treat the common cold. The seeds are said to "increase the milk in women's breasts" All this nourishment makes borage an excellent culinary herb. It is most valuable for those on salt-free diets, and when the young cucumber-flavoured leaves are chopped very finely to break down the soft hairs, they are excellent in salads and sandwiches. The larger leaves, too, must be chopped and they can be used in a strained, prepared soup stock which is simmered with the lid on (to retain the valuable essences) then put in batches into a blender and pureed. There will be no sign of the bristly hairs, they will be softened in the cooking. If serving hot, reheat the soup and serve with a blue borage flower on top. It is also delicious eaten icy cold in summer, garnished in the same way. The azure flowers are edible and may be used to decorate a green salad after tossing, floated on punches, or in individual glasses. Crystallised borage flowers are very pretty for decorating cakes and desserts, like crystallised violets, rose petals and mint leaves.

Medicinal – Because of all the wonderful health-giving properties contained in this plant, borage has a significant place in herbal medicine. It has been used as a heart tonic and to stimulate the adrenal glands. An old saying is: "I, Borage, bring always courage" Another herbalist of old says: "Those of our time do use the flour in sallads, to exhilerate and make the mind glad. There be also many things made of them, used for the comfort of the heart, to drive away sorrow". Compresses of the leaves have been used to relieve congested veins in the legs. The herb is still taken to help dispel excess watery elements from the body, as well as having a soothing effect on the digestion. French herbalists use it for colds, fevers, bronchitis, and for treating rheumatism.

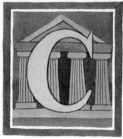

CARAWAY

(*Carum carvi*) Umbelliferae
Biennial

It is often thought that caraway is a spice rather than a herb because of the widespread use of its dried seeds, which are generally classified among the spices. The foliage and roots also have their culinary and medicinal uses, and it can be grown with other herbs in the garden. Propagation is by seed in a sheltered, sunny position in medium-textured, well-drained soil that is not arid or sandy. Germination is sometimes disappointing, with perhaps only one or two plants resulting from a seed packet. Seedlings are available from herb nurseries at the right time of year (late spring and summer), which usually is more satisfactory than starting from "scratch". Caraway can grow to 60 cm (2 ft), with feathery foliage and summer-blooming, pink-tinged, white parsley-type flowers. Let the blooms fade and the petals fall so that the tiny crescent-moon seeds can form: when they turn toast-brown, pluck the heads before all the seed has fallen, and sift the husks out. Store seeds in an airtight container. Cut the spent flower stems to ground level, so that the plant will grow up again in its second year.

Caraway is indigenous to several countries including Europe, North Africa and Asia. The ancient Egyptians, Romans and Greeks knew of its therapeutic qualities, and it is surrounded with mystique, including the belief that love potions containing caraway will keep the loved one from straying!

In astrology it is classified as a "mercurial" plant, and in companion planting it does not like fennel, each herb inhibiting the growth and full potential of the other.

Uses:

Culinary – Caraway seed, like aniseed, fennel, dill and coriander, contains aromatic oils that the plant's natural alchemy has distilled from the sun's rays. Chewing the seeds will help to dispel flatulence and improve the digestion. Used in cooking, it will help to digest foods that could otherwise create flatulence or lie heavily in the stomach. Caraway seed cake is traditional in England, and equally traditional in Holland and Germany is its inclusion in breads, rolls, certain cheeses, some confectionery, and in cabbage dishes. The liqueur Kummel has oil of caraway as its base. Certain vegetables, such as baked onions (or in a sauce for boiled onions), beetroot and carrots, are assimilated more easily if a few caraway seeds are mixed into them during cooking. If steaming cabbage, turnips, or parsnips, sprinkle a few seeds over the vegetables during cooking. If baking apples or pears, shake some seeds over them for a change of flavour and to help the digestion. Some people dislike the taste of caraway, so use aniseed, dill seed or fennel seed instead. The leaves and roots of caraway also have their uses because they contain similar nutritional and healing values. Young leaves are deliciously spicy in green salads, added to spinach during cooking, and to soups during the last half hour on the stove. The roots may be sliced and steamed and finished with a sauce, or melted butter, and eaten as a vegetable.

Medicinal – All parts of caraway assist the activity of the glands and kidneys. Most of caraway's medicinal properties lie in the potency of the seeds, which are even said to sharpen the eyesight when taken internally. The ground seeds, or the essential oil from them, is used today in medicines to help dispel flatulence, to aid the digestion, and to rid the body of excess fluids. The processed seed is also part of many other medicines.

Culpeper says the boiled roots, eaten like parsnips, strengthen the digestion of elderly people.

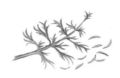

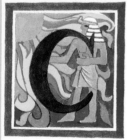

CHAMOMILE

(Anthemis nobilis) Compositae
Perennial

There are many different species of chamomile, all with similar small, daisy-like blossoms, usually single, with various properties: some, like the white blooming pyrethrum *Chrysanthemum cinerariifolium,* are insect repellents, and their potent flowers are used in natural garden sprays obtainable from nurseries, particularly those specialising in herbs. Another interesting chamomile, *C. parthenium,* is found in old gardens because it self-sows easily; it has either green or gold foliage, with white petal-rays surrounding the central yellow floret, and is known as "feverfew" or "febrifuge". Although it is sometimes used medicinally, it is not considered to be as therapeutically effective as German chamomile.

English chamomile *(Anthemis nobilis)* is a perennial and is grown as a ground cover because of its attractive, matting, feathery leaves. It does not flower as profusely as the German chamomile *(Matricaria chamomilla),* although the white, yellow-centred daisy-like flowers are sometimes used in chamomile teas, and when it is grown as an emerald-green lawn it looks charming, especially when starred with blooms here and there. It is best grown in broken sunlight or in a shady area in light soil and should be watered regularly with the sprinkler left on for an hour or two, unless the climate is fairly cold, with frequent drizzly rain. The most successful species of chamomile for a lawn is *Anthemus treneague,* but it is very difficult to obtain. English chamomile is propagated from seed or by root division. When in flower it grows to 30 cm (12 inches). Both English and German chamomile bloom from spring through autumn.

German chamomile is happier living in the sun than is the English chamomile, and it also likes to grow in light soil. Propagation is by seed only, and when in flower it reaches a height of 45–60 cm (1–1½ ft). It blooms prolifically and is the best species for herb teas. Gathering the flower heads is fairly demanding: the tiny white flowers, smaller than those of English chamomile, must be observed daily. The green immature centres are composed of minuscule golden petals which, when fully open, are the size of a pin-head. The flowers should not be plucked until the green centres have turned yellow because this is the most potent part of the herb. When they are ready, cut off the heads, using scissors. This must be done early in the morning, preferably by 10 a.m. Dry them by spreading them out on sheets of clean paper in the shade, or on a sieve. When dry, store in clean, airtight containers. Harvesting of the flowers continues right through the season, as more appear all the time. A very knowledgeable agricultural herbalist told us that if the flowers are picked after 10 a.m., or 12 noon, at the latest: "You may as well throw them away!" The sun is at its peak at midday and all the etheric energies of the plant are drawn upwards and will dissipate into the air; after 12 o'clock, the life-force of the plant starts to recede towards the root as the sun moves from its zenith, until by evening the vitality is concentrated in the roots. This is why replanting should be done late in the day, when the plants are stronger and better able to withstand the move.

Culpeper wrote that the Egyptians dedicated chamomile to the sun.

Uses:

Culinary – Chamomile foliage is nutritious and a small amount, snipped or chopped finely, gives an aromatic, peppery flavour to a tossed green salad, and stimulates the appetite. A few fresh flowers, which also are edible, can be strewn over the salad before serving. Chamomile tea is made by steeping the flowers in boiling water for a few minutes. It is then strained, resulting in a pleasant and fruity-tasting drink not unlike the flavour of pineapple juice. Sweeten with honey if you like but do not add milk. In summer, a stronger brew can be made which, when cooled, can be stored in the refrigerator: when ready to serve, pour into a jug filled with sparkling mineral water and serve as a delicious, nutritious cold drink. Add ice cubes and thin slices of lemon.

Medicinal – Chamomile contains a natural volatile oil, a glucosade and some tannic acid. The tea has been known and respected for centuries as being soothing and calming, German chamomile being the most effective. In Europe many people take it as their customary "night-cap" to relax them before going to bed. *A few drops only,* added occasionally to a baby's bottle of milk, will help calm and settle a restless infant. The quantities recommended for making herb teas (see p. 89) may be taken by older children during study time, or when under stress; exam students and tired businessmen benefit from a cup of chamomile tea at the end of the day. This tea is also a time-honoured potion to relieve menstrual pain. A strong infusion of the tea is excellent poured into a night-time bath to help relax and soothe tired muscles. Another remarkable quality of this herb is its ability to cure sties. Make a tea, pour through a *very fine strainer,* soak a piece of cotton wool in the lukewarm liquid and apply to the sty three times during the day. The sty should have almost disappeared by the end of the first day. A customer who visited our herb shop told us about this simple remedy and we have used it ourselves with great success. Chamomile tea when cooled, is also an excellent hair rinse. Used regularly for a few weeks, it adds highlights to the hair and makes naturally blond hair even fairer.

Chamomile in the garden is a "healer", helping sickly trees, shrubs and other plants that are close by.

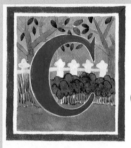

CHERVIL
(Anthriscus cerefolium) Umbelliferae
Annual

Chervil is a spicy-tasting herb with delicately cut foliage resembling fine, green lace. It is propagated by seed in spring, and where winters are mild, in autumn as well. Where summers are very hot it likes semi-shade and frequent watering. In winter it thrives in sunlight, even for only half a day. Our chervil bed in the herb garden happens to be in an ideal spot. It is partly shaded in summer and exposed to much more light in winter – the sun being angled differently in these two seasons. If you have a sheltered spot in your garden where the conditions are similar, put your chervil there, otherwise you could grow it under a deciduous tree that has a thin leaf cover so that the plants will have broken sunlight and air in summer, and in winter, when the leaves have fallen, the sunshine will filter through the bare branches. Chervil prefers average, moist soil. Its normal height when fully grown is 30 cm (12 inches). The white parsley-type flowers appear in early spring, and, in warm climates in autumn too. When the blooms have faded and produced seed, if allowed to fall they will usually germinate, especially during drizzly weather or if the surface is kept moist. However, if you wish to be certain of germination, collect the seeds when ripe, and plant them in soil that has been finely dug over and enriched with some compost

or a little poultry manure. You will soon be rewarded with another crop.

Chervil was a favourite of the Romans, who took the herb with them (amongst many others) wherever they created new homes in the lands they occupied. It is a nutritious and flavoursome addition to food, and has medicinal properties as well. On the Continent it is customary to serve chervil soup on Holy Thursday. It has also confusingly been called sweet cicely (Myrrhis odorata), which it resembles. Another herb bearing a close likeness to chervil is hemlock (Conium maculatum), a poisonous, though medicinal herb which should not be taken unless prepared correctly by a herbal medicine practitioner.

Astrologers agree that chervil is ruled by Jupiter.

Uses:
Culinary – There are four culinary herbs which make a choice and savoury bouquet called fines herbes, the others being tarragon, parsley and chives, and sometimes lemon thyme as well. When finely chopped and mixed in equal proportions they flavour and garnish omelettes, herb sandwiches to accompany soups or entrées, and add fragrance to green salads. Sprinkle over cooked chicken and fish, or fold into a sauce to accompany them. Stir into seafood or poultry mornays. In fact, the blend is not meant to flavour and embellish

robust-tasting food, its role is to subtly enhance the flavour of otherwise
bland dishes. Chervil on its own may
be used in the same way as *fines herbes*.
It should be added either at the end of
the cooking time or about five minutes before. Two or three teaspoons
(or more) of the chopped leaves may
be stirred into scrambled eggs, cream
cheese, mashed potato, and into a
smooth sauce. To make chervil soup,
use as a base a mixture of puréed vegetables and chicken stock, and stir in a
generous quantity of the finely chopped green leaves just before serving.

Medicinal – In spring, the leaves of
chervil have traditionally been eaten to
purify the blood and to rid the body of
excess fluids. It is said to stimulate the
glands and to benefit the kidneys. It
also relieves rheumatism and gout. An
old remedy was to apply a warm chervil poultice to painful joints. It is
believed to have rejuvenating qualities
and to act as a tonic. The volatile oil
extracted from the plant has a similar
aroma to myrrh.

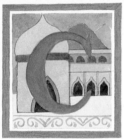

CHICORY

(Cichorium intybus) Compositae
Perennial

Chicory is a herb with a number of nutritional and medicinal qualities. When young, the long, broad leaves are at first bunched together in a clump, like spinach or sorrel, and then as the plant grows it sends out many branching stems with tiny, sparsely scattered leaves, finally achieving a height of 1.80 m (6 ft) or more. In midsummer the buds burst open revealing sky-blue, single, starry blooms which furl again at noon; on dull days they remain open all day. The finely serrated petals radiate from navy-blue central stamens; bees visit the flowers constantly when they are open. Seed is sown in spring, and the plants will grow almost anywhere but prefer average, well-drained soil and a sunny position.

The leaves and roots of the plant are used; the root being a coffee substitute or additive. The roots and the indented foliage at the base of the plant resemble dandelions in flavour, use and therapeutic properties. The leaves also yield a blue dye.

Chicory is known by several names and is called witloof or Belgian endive in its cultivated form. For this, young plants are forced in the dark and are prepared in a special way for blanching and compressing the leaves into tightly folded, elongated, creamy coloured heads; blanching also reduces excess bitterness. In England, the old name for chicory was succory and in many country areas it is still known by this name.

Historians agree that chicory is native to Europe and that it was known to the ancient Egyptians, Greeks, Arabians and Romans, who also knew how to blanch the leaves.

Astrologers say it is a plant under Jupiter.

Uses: *Culinary* – Blanched chicory, known as witloof or Belgian endive, is a sought-after delicacy and can be eaten raw or lightly cooked and prepared in different ways. Added to a green salad the crisp leaves give it a tantalising flavour. It is characteristically bitter, although the whiter and younger the leaves, the less bitter they are. Experienced cooks choose the fattest, firmest and creamiest of heads, even if some of the outside leaves are fringed with pale gold; but if the fringing is green and on several of the leaves and the heads feel limp, do not buy it.

For a green salad, carefully pull whole leaves from the tight head, wash them, dry well, and leave to crisp up in the refrigerator. For a salad on its own, either prepare the leaves in the same way and toss them in a French dressing, or cut the whole washed head either into circles, lengthways, or slantways, before tossing. To cook, cut the head in half lengthways, simmer or steam gently until just tender, drain and serve hot, masked with a favourite sauce. It can also be cut into smaller pieces and mixed into the sauce instead. Another good way to serve chicory is to steam small whole heads, or halved if larger, then drain, wrap ham around them, cover with sauce, perhaps add a little grated cheese, and grill until golden. The tender young green leaves can be freshly picked and added to a salad; but be warned, they are bitter, although not unpleasantly so, especially if eaten in moderation or mixed with other fresh, leafy greens. Young dandelion leaves can be eaten in the same way. While enjoying chicory as a food, it is good to know that it is extremely good for the liver as well as being a blood purifier and an appetiser.

Medicinal – The roots are used more often in herbal medicine than the leaves because they contain the greatest healing properties. The roots, dried and ground, are sometimes added to coffee, or a coffee-type beverage. The root has laxative properties and also helps rid the body of excess fluid. Like the leaves, the root is excellent for liver complaints and helps the flow of bile. A decoction made from the root is also used for rheumatic conditions and gout.

Culpeper says that the juice, or bruised leaves, mixed with a little vinegar, reduces swellings and inflammations when applied externally. Parkinson, another olden-day herbalist of esteem, declared chicory to be a "fine, cleansing, jovial plant". Chicory should not be taken too often or too freely because it is said to cause congestion of the digestive organs, but used in moderation it can do no harm.

Chicory greens are very good fodder for some animals, including sheep, cows and horses.

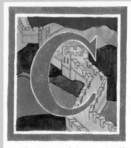

CHIVES

(*Allium schoenoprasum* Liliaceae
Perennial

Onion chives *(Allium schoenoprasum)* have been cultivated for thousands of years in nearly every country of the ancient world. It is said that the Chinese used chives in about 3000 B.C. and it was a favourite herb in Mediterranean lands before the Christian era. The great Emperor Charlemagne, in A.D. 812, listed chives among more than 70 other herbs for his gardens. Their use in Britain is said to have begun in the Middle Ages. Propagation is by seed in spring (also autumn in mild climates) and by division of the bulbs. Chives like fairly rich, well-drained soil in a sunny position and grow to 30 cm (12 inches). The leaves shrivel and die in midwinter and sprout again shortly afterwards from their bulbs, which increase each season. If left, the clump can become overgrown and the plants will not thrive, so divide them when they look starved and crowded. The mauve, pin-cushion summer blossoms have fine, stiff stalks which should be cut from the base; a mass of flowers will reduce the strength of the plants. To collect seed for re-sowing, allow some of the blooms to bear, then gather the seed before cutting off the stems. If you like onions but are worried about the effect on your breath, chives have

an onion flavour but leave no trace of odour. Chives should be picked from the base of the outside of the clump, allowing new shoots to mature from the centre. Use your fingers to pick chives because cutting with scissors will result in the top few centimetres turning hay-coloured and unattractive.

Garlic chives, or Chinese chives *(A. tuberosum)* look like onion chives when they germinate, and young tufts of thin, green shoots will appear. As the plant grows the foliage changes shape and becomes flat and long with a distinct garlic flavour. When fully grown they are 60 cm (2 ft) high; the clustered heads of white, green-centred starry blooms are carried on strong, upstanding stems. Cut these stalks at the base to maintain the strength of the plant, or let some go to seed and collect for re-sowing. They do not die away like onion chives.

Culpeper says that chives are under the dominion of Mars and that "they are indeed a kind of leeks, hot and dry in the fourth degree".

Uses:
Culinary – The delicate onion taste of chives complements the subtle bouquet of *fines herbes,* together with chopped parsley, chervil and tarragon in equal parts: each of these herbs is

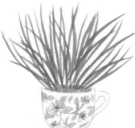

light and lingeringly aromatic in different ways, making a perfectly balanced blend of flavours. Chives on
their own flavour food when onions
would be too obtrusive. Although
chives contain a certain amount of a
pungent, volatile, sulphurous oil, pre-
sent in varying degrees in all the leek
family, from which it comes, there is
less in chives than in onions, making
them easier to digest. Chopped chives
can be used to garnish and flavour
omelettes, cooked poultry and fish,
salads, herb sandwiches, soups, mornays, and steamed, buttered vegetables. They add flavour to all kinds of
savoury sauces, mayonnaise and
cream cheese.

Garlic chives are coarser than onion
chives and should be chopped very
finely before using them. Always add
both onion chives and garlic chives
during the last few minutes of cooking
otherwise their delicate flavour will be
destroyed. If you are a garlic devotee,
garlic chives can be added to scrambled eggs, omelettes, mashed cream
cheese, herb sandwiches, and in all the
ways you would use onion chives.
One memorable afternoon tea, taken
with a dear friend, was our favourite
Earl Grey tea, poured from a silver
teapot, with one simple accompaniment – chopped garlic chives on cream
cheese and butter, spread between
thinly sliced crustless fresh bread cut
into triangles, and served on a snowy
napkin in a gleaming silver dish.
Medicinal – Chives, like many other
herbs, contain calcium, which strengthens nails and teeth. Chives also stimulate the appetite and tone up the kidneys. They assist in lowering high
blood pressure.

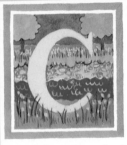

COMFREY

(Symphytum officinalis) Boraginaceae
Perennial

Comfrey is a herb with powerful therapeutic properties. A native of Europe and parts of temperate Asia, it is found growing wild in damp places such as river banks, ditches, streams and water meadows. It belongs to the same family as borage and forget-me-not. Propagation is by seed, which is difficult, as its germination is sometimes unreliable. We have sown it straight into prepared trays from seed heads from our own plants with no results at all, but this may have been just bad luck, or the seed may not have been quite ready. The surest way of increasing the plant is by root division or root cuttings, and it propagates itself by sending up new plants from its root system. Spring (and autumn in mild climates) is the time for propagation. When it is ready to plant out, choose a shady, moist place, or keep the seedlings watered if the bed is dry. It grows to 1.20 m (4 ft), and the parts used are the leaves and roots. In summer the mauve flowers grow in pendulous bunches at the ends of their stems. The outside broad leaves can grow to an enormous length, sometimes up to 60 m (2 ft). The stalks and foliage are hairy, although not prickly like borage. Garden predators such as caterpillars, snails and slugs are particularly fond of comfrey and unless you keep a constant watch on the plants, these pests will munch into the

leaves until they resemble fine lace, or will leave unsightly holes and rents in the leaves. To help keep them away, use a natural spray, or powder the dampened leaves lightly twice a week with derris dust, an old, well-tried, non-chemical insecticide extracted from plants. There is another type of comfrey, known as "Russian comfrey", which is highly regarded as a fodder plant.

Recently, scientific experiments on laboratory rats has shown that taking comfrey in large amounts can cause cancer (because of a component in the plant). Historically, however, comfrey has had an undisputed place in herbal medicine for thousands of years; in fact to many it has been almost a "miracle" herb. The Romans knew its value in helping to mend broken bones and its country name, even to this day, is "knitbone". The scientific name of *symphytum* is thought to come from the Greek word *symphyo* which, loosely translated, means "to make whole".

That keen old astrologer, Dr Culpeper, says that comfrey is "a herb of Saturn and under the sign of Capricorn, cold, dry and earthy in quality".

Uses:
Culinary – The tender young leaves, with the fresh taste of cucumber, make an agreeable addition to a green salad. The older leaves tend to be

tough when raw and are not as pleasant to eat. A favourite way of cooking the young leaves is to coat them in batter and fry them gently in oil; they are eaten hot with a little pepper and salt, as a vegetable. Any slight hairiness on the foliage disappears when comfrey is cooked. Chopped fresh comfrey leaves added to spinach while cooking makes it even more nutritious. When cooked on its own, comfrey becomes glutinous, but when some of the chopped leaves are added to chicken stock and simmered, and then puréed in a blender, this is not so noticeable. *Medicinal* – Comfrey contains vitamin B 12 and calcium as well as allantoin, giving it the ability to help in healing broken bones and wounds as well as maintaining strong teeth. Taken as a tea it is soothing and healing and good for the circulation. If you prefer to use comfrey externally, a poultice made from the root and leaves is recommended by herbalists for wounds and fractures. Comfrey ointment or cream has great soothing and healing properties for the skin, and a friend with a perfect complexion uses nothing else as a night cream after removing her make-up with apricot kernel oil. Comfrey ointment is also used to rub into painful rheumatic joints. Comfrey leaves made into a tea for a facial steam help to freshen and tighten tired and ageing skins.

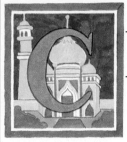

CORIANDER

(Coriandrum sativum) Umbelliferae

Annual

Coriander belongs to a large tribe of herbs, all with the same type of spreading, delicate flower heads as parsley, hence the generic name of Umbelliferae, which aptly describes the umbrella-shaped formation of the blooms. The colours of the flowers vary in this family, those of coriander being white, faintly tinged with pale lavender.

Propagation is by seed (which stays viable for seven years), in spring, and again in autumn in temperate climates. Sow straight into prepared beds containing broken-up, fine soil in a well-drained, sunny, sheltered position. The plants will grow to 45-60 cm (1½-2 ft), or even higher if the aspect and season are especially favourable. We had a group of about a dozen that grew to 1.20 m (4 ft); covered in their fairy-floss flowers, they looked especially enchanting amongst their green-lace foliage. If your plants grow fairly high, tie them to thin bamboo stakes to protect them from winds which may damage the slender stalks.

The leaves, with their finely cut margins, resemble chervil or anise but the flavour is distinctly different and individual. At first bite, the unique taste is strongly aromatic and, to some, not appealing. When used in discreet amounts, coriander leaves can

lift an ordinary dish into something quite memorable. It is often referred to as Chinese parsley and appears extensively in Oriental cooking. The seeds, or fruit, are also extremely useful and they, too, have a pungency and taste that is quite different from any other herb or spice.

As the flower goes to seed, the fruits which follow are bright green at first and have the same flavour as the leaves, but when the seeds are ready for harvesting and turn a light fawn colour, the flavour subtly changes to deliciously aromatic; they are described in the Bible as "like wafers made with honey" (Exodus 16.31). This is the time to remove the heads and put them in a box to dry; they can even be exposed to some sunlight for a few hours to complete the drying process. When the seeds start to fall, give the heads a final shake into the box, and sift the coriander through a sieve to remove any husks, then store in an airtight jar.

Coriander is native to southern Europe from where it has found its way to other parts of the world. It grows wild in Britain and is also widely grown in China, Peru, India and the Middle East. Dr Culpeper does not mention coriander in his *Herbal,* so we do not

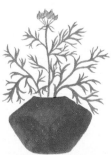

know which astrological sign it comes under.

Uses:

Culinary – Coriander leaves are an essential ingredient in many of the regional dishes of the countries where it is grown, for instance in Asian, Middle Eastern and Indian food. The pretty leaves also make an attractive garnish. Coriander leaves are becoming popular in European cooking and when used carefully they enhance the flavour of certain dishes. Ground coriander seed is popular and is one of the main ingredients of curries and other mixed spice dishes. The ground seed is used to flavour all kinds of food, from fish, poultry and meat to cakes, biscuits, bread, and some vegetables, such as eggplant (aubergine), zucchini (courgettes), capsicums and mushrooms. It can also be dusted over apples, pears or peaches while baking, giving them a piquant flavour. When left whole, the seed is also an ingredient in pickling spice mixtures.

Medicinal – Coriander was among the herbs mentioned in the *Medical Papyrus of Thebes* written in 1552 B.C.

It was valued by Hippocrates in classical Greek medicine, and in nutrition and medicine by the Arabs and Hebrews. The seeds have much the same properties as dill, caraway and fennel in that they help to disperse flatulence. Like other fruits of this genus, the seeds are high in valuable constituents, coriander yielding a percentage of a pale yellow volatile oil, the active ingredient, as well as malic acid and tannin. Coriander is also a stimulant and is often used in commercial medicines as a flavouring and to counteract the griping pains caused by some aperients. Coriander was prescribed for treating kidney stones, and for purifying the blood. Convalescents in some European countries were given a soup made from barley water and coriander leaves as a recuperative tonic.

It has been warned that the seeds can become narcotic if taken too often.

Whole or ground coriander seed added to a potpourri mixture gives it a soft, warm and spicy scent.

Bees love coriander flowers, and chervil and coriander grown together make good companion plants.

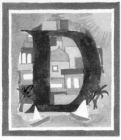

DILL

(Anethum graveolens) Umbelliferae

Annual

Dill originated from Mediterranean lands and southern Russia, even though the herb has been naturalised for centuries in many other countries, and is seen growing wild along roadsides and in fields where conditions are suitable. At first sight the ferny appearance of the foliage makes it difficult to distinguish dill from fennel, but on closer inspection it can be noticed that fennel's leaves are a light, bright green colour, and when biting into a feathery leaf the flavour and aroma are reminiscent of licorice or aniseed. Dill is more fragile looking, the foliage almost a blue-green, and the flavour of the leaves is distinctive, much "dryer", and slightly peppery and spicy.

Seed may be sown in spring (and autumn in mild climates) in a sunny, sheltered position in light, well-drained soil. When in flower in spring and summer, it is 90 cm (3 ft) in height. The pale yellow blooms are typically umbelliferous in shape, spreading and expanded like an open umbrella. Each flower head is made up of about 24 wiry stalks, the outer ones being longer than those in the middle, carrying approximately 20 minute florets, each one on the tiniest stem imaginable. Pick a floret on its thin stalk from the composite bloom and see how like a fairy bouquet it is. When the flower head has dropped its petals, oval flat seeds will have

formed. For harvesting, cut the heads and lay them in a box, sun-dry them for a few hours, then shake out all the seeds and sieve them to remove the husks. Store in an airtight, labelled container.

In the garden, dill is helpful to certain plants in the vegetable patch: corn, lettuce and cucumber, for instance. Bees are attracted to the pollen-laden flowers.

The herbal and astrological specialist, Dr Culpeper, says: "Mercury has dominion over this plant and therefore it strengthens the brain".

Uses:

Culinary – The pungent taste of dill leaves makes them an excellent flavouring for almost any food. Try dill instead of parsley sometimes. When finely chopped, the leaves are delicious in mashed potatoes, cream cheese, white sauce, omelettes, any fish or shellfish dishes, salads, soups, cooked buttered vegetables, and as a flavouring for vinegar. The chopped leaves are delicious when spread over lamb, veal or chicken when roasting, with more stirred into the gravy before serving. The leaves, and sometimes the flowers and seeds as well, are used to make "dill pickles".

Although dill leaves have some valuable constituents, there is greater nutritional and medicinal value in the seeds. Dill seeds, or fruit, like other umbelliferous seeds, contain volatile oils which are stimulating to the system, disperse flatulence, and are also soothing to the nerves. Dill seed can be added to gas-forming vegetables such as cabbage, when making sauerkraut, coleslaw, or steaming it as a vegetable, to make it easier to digest. They can also be used with cucumbers, onions, and some root vegetables, as well as pastries, breads, and some sauces.

Medicinal – Dill water helps soothe and calm babies who are troubled with flatulence and is a very old remedy going back to the days of the Norse peoples. (Dill is also said to have properties which strengthen the fingernails.) Oil of dill is sold by some chemists for digestive upsets: suck a sugar cube with a few drops of the oil added to it. Dill soup, made from the leaves, chicken stock and egg yolks, is nutritional and delicious.

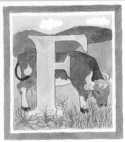

FENNEL

(Foeniculum vulgare dulce) Umbelliferae
Annual

Florence fennel, also known as sweet fennel and finocchio fennel, is the best variety to use in food. We have also read of other types of fennel growing in many countries, variously called Saxon fennel, Russian and Roumanian fennel, French bitter fennel, Roman fennel, Sicilian fennel, Indian fennel and Japanese fennel. Two kinds that we have seen, besides Florence fennel, are bronze-leaved fennel, whose foliage is dark and bronze-coloured and is edible, and of course the wild, tall variety *(F. vulgare)* that grows everywhere. The latter is a perennial and its leaves are edible, the flavour being coarser and ranker than sweet fennel. All parts of Florence fennel may be used. It originally came from the Mediterranean countries, and was part of Greek mythology.

Propagation is by seed in spring (in autumn too where winters are not very severe, and it is the autumn sowing that is effective for cultivating the bulbous base to large proprotions, even though there will be some swelling at other times). The soil should be medium to light and well drained. When fully grown it is 90 cm (3 ft) high, or taller. The swollen stem base is a sought-after delicacy, the aromatic leaves are especially good with fish, and the seeds, like those of dill and caraway, have digestive properties. The

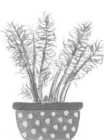

flower heads, which bloom in spring, are similar to dill but are a brighter gold in colour, and more prolific. The plant itself is covered in luxurious plumes of light, green foliage, every graceful leaf being made up of hair-thin, aromatic fronds borne on sappy stems. The seed, or fruit, forms when the flower has dropped its petals; they are fatter than dill seeds and crop well. They should be dried and stored as for dill seeds. To make the most of fennel's swollen base, the plant needs plenty of water, it should be fed with well-decayed poultry manure and the earth hilled up around the area. This treatment should be continued for about fourteen days, then the base should be sliced away from the roots, washed well, and the foliage removed. Do not throw away the leaves, wrap them in foil or plastic film and store them in the refrigerator.

Fennel should not be planted with caraway, coriander, wormwood, tomatoes, kohlrabi and beans. Fennel helps to repel fleas and when used to supplement the feed of cows and goats, will increase their milk supply.

Culpeper says Mercury is fennel's star sign. He has quite a lot to say of its many benefits in medicine, although the remedy that appeals most is his advice to the overweight: "Both leaves, seeds, and roots thereof, are much used in drink or broth, to make people lean that are too fat".

Uses:

Culinary – A few finely chopped fennel leaves will add flavour to potato salad, green salad, spaghetti and rice, and will help to digest them. It is traditional to cook fennel leaves with oily fish to help cut the richness: make incisions in the fish if grilling, and push small fennel fronds into each cut. Another method is to butter or oil a baking dish, make a bed of leafy fennel branches and place the fish on top. Add a little more oil or butter, and salt and pepper if you like, and some thinly sliced lemon, and bake in a moderate oven until cooked. The leaves will become brittle and brown, and a few will cling to the fish, so there is no need to serve the layer of singed fennel as well because the fish itself will be delicately permeated with the flavour.

The swollen stem base, tasting crisp and fragrant with a fine texture (seen in greengrocers' shops during winter), can be sliced thinly, the pieces separated and mixed into a green salad, or served as a salad on its own with French dressing.

"Finocchio" can be sliced either vertically or horizontally. The base, cut in half, steamed, and covered with white sauce, makes an excellent vegetable; or prepare a light meal with a cheese sauce poured over the cooked, halved fennel bulbs, adding some chopped fennel leaves and parsley, and then baking until golden-brown.

The seeds, whole or ground, are nutritious too, and help digest starchy foods like bread, pastries and pasta. As with dill and caraway, they reduce flatulence when used with cabbage dishes, Brussels sprouts, broccoli, cauliflower and onions. Ground fennel seeds are also mixed with other spices to flavour curries.

Medicinal – Fennel roots, although not considered as effective as the seeds, were also used in medicine. The volatile oil expressed from the fruit (or seeds) is excellent for dispelling flatulence and it is used in herbal laxatives to relieve colicky pains. A tea made from the seeds helps to dispel gas, rids the body of excess fluids, and aids the digestion generally. Fennel seed tea, well strained, bathes sore eyes: this infusion is well known in folk medicine as being beneficial to the eyesight. The pleasant fragrance of fennel oil is often used commercially when making cordials and liqueurs, some perfumery and soaps.

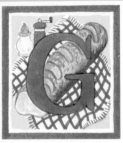

GARLIC

(Allium sativum) Liliaceae
Perennial

Aromatic garlic is a herb that has been known and valued in nutrition and medicine since antiquity. It is thought to have originated in south-eastern Siberia and spread from there to ancient Egypt, Greece, Italy and other countries. It is also mentioned in ancient Chinese writings.

The garlic bulb is composed of tightly clustered bulblets, or "cloves", and the plant is propagated, in spring, by these bulblets. Propagation by seed is not recommended; it is slow and not always reliable. Plant the curved segment with its root-end down in a sunny, well-drained position in previously dug and manured soil. Press each bulblet into drills 5 cm (2 inches) deep, cover with more soil and lightly firm down. It is a good idea to plant several in a row, keeping them 15 cm (6 inches) apart. Do not let the ground dry out, a little watering each day is needed if there is no rain or drizzle. The segments will soon send up pale green flat leaves and the plants are usually ready to harvest in about six months, when the bulbs should be dug up.

Garlic flowers look like a giant chive flower, although the colour is creamy rather than mauve. When the flowers have begun to fade and the leaves start to turn yellow and to shrivel, the bulbs are mature enough to harvest. Dig

them up, shake off the excess soil, slice off the long roots, plait the remaining leaves clinging to the top of the bulbs and hang them in a dry, airy place. When the knobs of garlic have hardened, remove any remaining foliage and store where the air can circulate around them, otherwise they will become mildewed. A large, open-weave basket makes an excellent storage place.

There are several varieties of garlic; the smooth, transparent skins that cover the bulbs differ in colour from white, to pink, and mauve. The flavour varies in the degree of pungency as well. We were once given a "Belgian garlic" which developed a bulb the size of a cricket ball with no segments; it was mild in flavour with a nutty texture.

In the garden, garlic is compatible with roses and helps to repel aphids. A garden spray made from crushed garlic cloves and other natural ingredients acts as an insect repellent. Certain commercial companies are now manufacturing garlic sprays which are obtainable from some nurseries.

Culpeper says that this powerfully flavoured herb is owned by Mars and that "... its head is vehement; and in choleric men it will add fuel to the fire. In men oppressed by melancholy, it

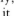

will attenuate the humour". He is also lavish in his praise of its many virtues for the betterment of health. This is equally true today.

Uses:

Culinary – Besides being a nutritious herb, it is also a necessity in the kitchen for flavouring many dishes. Before using, break off as many segments as will be needed, peel away the tissue-like covering, and then use it as directed in the recipe. Sometimes all you need to do is to rub a salad bowl, or a casserole dish, with a cut clove of garlic. A marvellous French Provincial mayonnaise, called *aioli,* is made with quantities of garlic crushed to a pulp, then made like a classic mayonnaise with beaten egg yolk and olive oil incorporated drop by drop. It is eaten as an accompaniment to globe artichokes, asparagus, steamed fish or poultry, snails or boiled potatoes.

It is said that if one eats garlic over a long period of time, the system assimilates its distinctive odours and they do not stay on the breath, or emanate from the pores of the skin.

Garlic is accepted as a flavouring in almost every country's cuisine, whether in recognisable amounts or in discreet quantities. It is paramount in regional Mediterranean dishes, and also goes well with lamb, pork, veal, beef, and curries. It brings out the flavour of tomatoes, eggplant (aubergine) and zucchini (courgettes). Garlic is used widely in Asian cooking, in many salads and certain sauces. Hot, garlic-flavoured bread is a favourite.

Medicinal – We are grateful to Clare Wilmot, a friend and brilliant naturopath and owner of The Triad Clinic in St Ives, New South Wales, for allowing us to quote her on garlic's many medicinal properties:

> Garlic contains the vitamins A, B, and C, and the elements copper, sulphur, manganese, iron and calcium, which make it valuable as a tonic for the cells and glands of the body. It has a particularly penetrative quality, which makes it a powerful antiseptic. When taken into the body, garlic helps to eliminate toxins from the bloodstream, stimulates the flow of bile and gastric juices, aids digestion, cleanses stale mucus from the tissues, nourishes the nerves, helps to prevent hardening of the arteries, increases glandular secretions and encourages the growth of healthful bacteria in the intestinal tract. It is therefore recognised as an important factor in promoting long life and maintaining health and youthful vigour.

Garlic contains a natural antibiotic substance and can be eaten raw or taken in capsule form. It is especially recommended for overseas travellers because it will help guard against infection. Eating garlic *au naturelle,* or taken in capsule form, is remarkably cleansing for the skin and banishes youthful pimples, prevents colds, soothes coughs and relieves sinus and bronchial troubles. Parsley is added to make odourless garlic capsules which are now available.

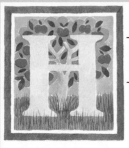

HORSERADISH

(Cochlearis armoracia) Cruciferae
Perennial

Horseradish is yet another herb that has been valued in food and medicine in many countries for thousands of years. It is said to be native to eastern Europe, and has become part of traditional cookery and medicine in many parts of the world. The extremely hot and pungent root is the part that is mainly used, although in the Middle Ages, the young leaves, as well as the root, were eaten.

Propagation is by root cuttings, or division, in spring. (The blooms set seed, but propagating from the roots is quicker.) Plant the rooted cuttings in rich, loose, moist soil in a shady position. Allow 30 cm (12 inches) between plants and keep them watered in dry weather. The green, slightly rough leaves are long and quite deeply indented. The flowers are white and have four cross-shaped petals that are typical of the Cruciferae family. They grow in tiny clusters on long stalks which spring from a main stem and have small leaf-spears underneath, appearing to support the flower stalks. The plant grows to approximately 90 cm (3 ft).

To collect the roots for use, scrape the soil away from the side of the plant and slice off one (or more) of the small roots, leaving the main one undisturbed. This can be done at any time once the plant is a reasonable

size. If you wish to harvest all the roots, they can be stored in dry sand. It is advisable to grow new plants either every year or every other year. This is not difficult because the root system is very strong and, if conditions are ideal, will produce new plants almost every year.

This herb, Dr Culpeper says, is "under Mars", and juice from the root was much used in his day to treat scurvy. A very diluted solution was given to children as a treatment for intestinal worms.

Horseradish in the garden is compatible with fruit trees and potatoes.

Uses:

Culinary – Horseradish root helps to digest rich and oily foods. For horseradish sauce the root is grated and combined with other ingredients, such as béchamel sauce, sour cream, thick fresh cream, or mayonnaise. Usually a little salt and sugar is added, together with a dash of vinegar or lemon juice and some mustard. A peeled, grated apple and some freshly chopped mint gives an unusual and refreshing flavour to the bitingly hot sauce. Horseradish sauce is served as an accompaniment to grilled, roasted or boiled beef, pork, ham, some fish and shellfish, and poultry. If you do not have a horseradish plant and find the fresh root difficult to obtain, dried horseradish is nearly always available in grocers' shops and is either powdered, granulated, or in flakes. Whichever you use, always give dried horseradish time to reconstitute once it is mixed with other ingredients; overnight or half a day should be enough. Freshly grated horseradish, or a little of the dried, gives a piquant tang to seafood sauces, mayonnaise, vinaigrette dressing, dips, spreads, and sour cream for baked potatoes. One or two of the young leaves, finely chopped, can be added to a green salad.

Medicinal – Horseradish root in the diet, or horseradish tablets, help to clear the sinuses and relieve nasal colds and bronchial complaints. Modern herbalists still use horseradish in specified doses as a digestive stimulant. It also acts as a diuretic and relieves rheumatism and gout. An ointment made from horseradish, rubbed on the chest, helps to disperse congestion from a cold. It is also said to assist in strengthening the blood vessels and in reducing blood pressure. The grated root can be mixed with yoghurt or milk and then patted on the skin (avoiding the eye area) to help fade freckles. The same solution can be used as a skin freshener.

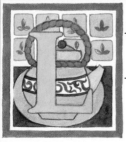

LEMON GRASS

(Cymbopogon citratus) Gramineae
Perennial

Lemon grass is a comparitive new-comer to our herb garden. It is a native of Asia, where it has been used for culinary and medicinal purposes for many years. Lemon grass is relatively unknown in European cooking and herbal medicine, but its delicate flavour and health-giving properties are becoming more widely recognised.

A friend and her husband, who is a Consul for one of the Asian countries, had just welcomed the new Ambassador to Australia. The strangers were to live in Canberra, the country's Federal Capital. The Ambassador's wife asked if she could have some lemon grass in the garden to remind her of home, and to use in cooking. At that time very few people had heard of it, and our lemon grass was originally given to us by an Indonesian couple who ran a restaurant. Our friend came to us hoping that we could help, and fortunately we were able to dig a sizeable slice from our well-established plant with plenty of soil clinging to the roots. Wrapped in damp sphagnum moss and a plastic bag, this parcel was taken to Canberra by our friends, much to the delight of the new diplomats.

A report several months later was ecstatic, the clump was doing well and had increased in size. We had a few doubts as to whether it would survive in the cold of a Canberra winter, but it did. If you live in an area where winters are cold and frosty, plant your lemon grass where it will receive sunshine for most of the day in a position where the roots can be kept moist. It does not like dry condition.

Lemon grass grows in a bushy clump, increasing in size each year. The roughish, narrow leaves bend gracefully outwards and have a slightly sticky texture. They are pale green and at certain times of the year are rust coloured at the tips. The foliage has a deliciously subtle lemon scent. In spring, the old leaves should be cut down to where the new shoots are appearing. From time to time during the year, if the plant is becoming spindly and ungainly, cut 15 cm (6 inches) off the tops of the leaves.

Propagation is by division of the roots. Dig well down into the ground with a spade, cutting cleanly through the main bush, and take as many clumps as you can without damaging the parent plant. Put the new shoots into prepared ground immediately, firm down the soil and water well. The ground is prepared by turning over the soil on the chosen site and making several drills ready to take the new lemon grass plants. We have not seen it flower during the many years that we have grown this herb.

Uses:

Culinary – Lemon grass is an ingredient that is very widely used in South-East Asian cooking. The tips, the tender shoots, and the leaves, cut off at ground level, are all used. It is particularly good in curries and other spicy dishes, when the stalks are used whole and then discarded before serving. Try snipping a few pieces of the leaf into a pot of tea for a refreshing, lemony flavour.

In European cooking, a bunch of lemon grass leaves put in the water when steaming or simmering a chicken, or fish, gives a delicate and delicious hint of lemon. The flavour of many other dishes can be enhanced by using the leaves in the same way.

Medicinal – Lemon grass oil contains vitamin A and, used externally, is beneficial for skin complaints. When taken as a tea, or in tablet form, it helps to clear the complexion, giving it a fine texture and healthy glow. Teenagers with skin problems will benefit from a course of lemon grass tablets, or by taking it as a tea. An extra bonus is that lemon grass taken in this way gives the eyes a bright, clear look. When a few drops of lemon grass oil are added to bathwater, the pores of the skin will open and absorb the essential elements from the oil.

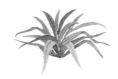

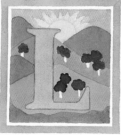

LOVAGE

(Levisticum officinalis) Umbelliferae
Perennial

Lovage is a herb that was highly thought of in ancient times but for some reason is not very widely used today. As well as being nutritious, it adds flavour to food and also has medicinal properties. It is a native of the mountainous areas of the Mediterranean region and was valued for its roots, stems, leaves and seeds, all of which give off an aromatic fragrance.

Propagation is by seed in spring, and it grows best in rich, moist soil in semi-shade. It reaches a height of 90 cm-1.5 m (3-5 ft) and bears a close resemblance to angelica. However, there are significant differences, lovage being a much smaller plant, and although the leaves are a similar shape, they are a fraction of the size of angelica leaves. The stems and stalks are hollow. The flavour of the foliage is peppery, and they are an excellent substitute for spices and pepper. The attractive yellow-green flowers bloom from midsummer to autumn and are typically umbelliferous in shape except that they are more closely clustered into a round composite form (similar to those of angelica) instead of spreading outward. The fruit or aromatic seeds are brown when ripe.

Culpeper says in astrology "It is an herb of the Sun under the sign of Taurus".

Uses: *Culinary –*
The chopped leaves give zest to soups, stews and casseroles, as well as to salads. It was known as a valued "pot-herb" in bygone days and was used in the same way, with other herbs and "weeds" gathered in their season. The leaves need to be cut up finely because of their slightly coarse texture. Add a few of the seeds and some of the sliced root for extra goodness and flavour. Although not as sweet, the hollow stems and stalks may be candied in the same way as angelica.

Medicinal – The curative powers of lovage are many and are chronicled by the old herbalists, much of their knowledge being still in use today. The plant has a high vitamin C content, and was popular for treating scurvy. The root is valuable for expelling flatulence and acts on the kidneys to rid the body of fluid waste during fevers. A tea made with the seeds is recommended by some herbal therapists as a gargle for throat infections, and as a drink for congestion of the lungs. The leaves, fresh or dried, infused as a tea or eaten raw in a salad or in sandwiches, act as a stimulant for the digestive organs. The strained tea also makes an excellent soothing lotion for sore eyes. Lovage also has deodorant properties, and a cooled lovage tea may be patted over the body with cotton wool. For a refreshing bath, make a very strong tea, or infusion, of the leaves, then strain into the bathwater.

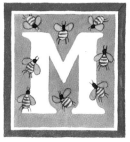

MARJORAM

(Origanum majorana) Labiatae
Perennial

Marjoram and oregano (sometimes called wild marjoram) belong to the *Origanum* family which is indigenous to the Mediterranean region but for centuries it has been widely distributed in Asia, North Africa, and other countries. Although the plants are very similar they have significant differences in flavour, leaf colour and texture, and innate robustness. Honey bees swarm around these bushes when in flower, and both these herbs have a beneficial effect on surrounding plants.

Dr Culpeper says that, astrologically, marjoram is a "a herb of Mercury under Aries" and that wild marjoram is also under the dominion of Mercury.

Marjoram seems to us to be a very "English" herb: it was used for strewing on floors in the days before carpets, rugs or mats were common, its sweet scent being released when trodden on. Furniture was often rubbed with marjoram leaves and it is still used as an ingredient in "sweet bags" or potpourris for linen cupboards and drawers.

Marjoram's leaves are velvet-soft, sweetly aromatic and a soft grey-green in colour. It is not as easy to rear as oregano and the plant is sometimes attacked by a disease called "damping-off". Those parts of the plant that are affected should be removed immediately.

Damping-off can be caused by unfavourable soil conditions or an unsuitable position.

Propagation is from seed or by cuttings in spring. Grow the plants in average, well-drained soil in a sunny position, with some shade in the afternoon during the hottest part of summer. It grows to 44 cm (1½ ft) and produces tiny, fluffy, pearly flowers in summer and autumn. There are a number of varieties of marjoram, but *O. majorana* is the easiest to obtain.

Uses:

Culinary – Marjoram, mixed with sage and thyme, forms the basic blend called simply 'mixed herbs'. When mixing the herbs, use one part each of marjoram and thyme to two parts of sage so as not to overpower the flavour of the marjoram. Sage has a completely different aroma and although pungent, has a dry, keen quality. Marjoram, on its own adds a subtle piquancy to salads, omelettes, sauces, scones and dumplings, and is also good in fish or poultry dishes and in clear soups. A few fresh, chopped or whole leaves scattered over buttered vegetables is also delicious. The soft whole leaves laid on a bed of cream cheese in herb sandwiches is another flavour treat.

Medicinal – Marjoram has been used to 'warm cold diseases of the head' and was extolled as an excellent remedy for the brain, bearing out the words of another old herbalist who said that to sniff marjoram frequently would ensure good health. The medicinal properties of the oil extracted from marjoram are almost identical to oregano oil. In modern herbal medicine, marjoram infused in hot water and sipped is excellent for nervous headaches and induces soothing sleep. It is also good for cramps and aids the digestion. When blended with chamomile it makes a tonic tea for the whole system. Marjoram oil can be gently rubbed into bruises and sprains and also relieves rheumatic pains. Like sage, it helps to darken the hair of brunettes, or those whose hair is turning grey. Fresh or dried marjoram leaves can be tied into a bag and added to bathwater. The dried leaves make a soothing and fragrant addition to a potpourri and to 'sleep pillows'.

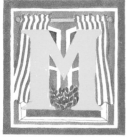

MINT

Labiatae
Annual

Mint is one of a number of herbs that orginated in the Mediterranean regions and it has been known and used since the earliest times. The Romans introduced it to Britain, and it is mentioned by Chaucer and Shakespeare in various works. In the Bible, the Pharisees were said to have been paid tithes of mint, amongst other herbs and spices. There are many different flavoured and unusual mints and their classification is becoming increasingly difficult because they cross-fertilise continually.

Spearmint *(Mentha spicata* or *M. viridis),* also called English mint, is the kind we know best. It has smooth, long, pointed leaves of bright green. Another species of spearmint, with exactly the same flavour and perfume although a hardier plant, has round, crinkled foliage of a slightly darker green and is variously called curly mint, common mint, garden mint or green mint.

Spearmint is propagated from seed, by cuttings, or by root division in spring. It prefers rich, moist soil in semi-shade or full shade. The white, clustered flowers grow together in a spear shape and mainly bloom in late summer to autumn when the plant grows to 30-90 cm (1-3 ft).

Culpeper says that astrologically it is a plant of Venus.

Peppermint *(M. piperita officinalas)* is an important medicinal herb and is cultivated mainly for its pungent, aromatic oil. It is not used in cooking but when taken as a tea it is highly therapeutic for many ailments.

Peppermint is propagated in the same way as spearmint, and it flowers at about the same time. The blooms are mauve and the leaves are purple-tinted. It grows to 30-90 cm (1-3 ft).

Culpeper claims it is a plant of Venus.

Pennyroyal *(M. pulegium)* is worth growing because it is a strong deterrent to mosquitos, especially when it is grown around barbecues and under bedroom windows. It also effectively repels fleas. A few green sprigs under the dog's mat will deter these insects, and if they invade the house, a few more sprigs in strategic places will help to get rid of them. Pennyroyal also has medicinal properties.

It is mainly propagated by root division and for most of the year it clings to the ground, every small tentacle having rootlets attached. Cuttings can be taken from these and replanted straightaway. In late summer it sends up spires of flower stalks, the blooms growing in lavender-coloured whorls up each stem. At this stage the plant reaches 30 cm (1 ft) in height. If growing pennyroyal as a lawn, mow the flowering stalks, or cut them off at the base, because if the plant is allowed to go to seed, it will spend itself. This minty herb, too, is under

Venus, according to the herbalist and astrologer, Dr Culpeper.

Eau-de-Cologne mint *(M. piperita citrata)* is worth cultivating for its delicious fragrance. It has dark green to purple-tinged leaves which may be added to fruit punches and cold summer drinks. The dried leaves are excellent in a potpourri mixture. Some of the mints that have become popular in recent years are apple mint or "Bowles mint" *(Mentha rotundifolia),* with round, apple-scented leaves; variegated apple mint with green and white leaves, which is a decorative variety and has a hint of sage. Others are pineapple mint, which has either plain green or variegated green and gold foliage; ground-hugging Corsican mint with diminutive, highly perfumed foliage; grey Japanese mint, which is not strongly scented; cardinal mint, which has a faint perfume of spearmint and smooth round leaves; Asian mint, a decorative variety with long-pointed neatly rounded leaves edged in dark red and tasting of hot chillies; licorice mint; ginger mint, which can have a yellow variegation, and basil mint, which is a good substitute for basil in winter when the real thing is not available.

Uses:

Culinary – Mint or spearmint is a time-honoured ingredient in mint sauce or mint jelly, which is traditionally eaten with lamb. It is also good cooked with peas; after draining the water, add a few more freshly chopped mint leaves and butter. Mint juleps are served in long, icy cold glasses with lavish circlets of fresh mint sprays around the rims. Chopped mint helps to make boiled baby new potatoes more digestible. Mint brings out the flavour of tomatoes and is a traditional ingredient in pea soup. When frying bananas for Chicken Maryland, first roll them in lemon juice and chopped mint. Whole mint leaves in green salads are delicious, especially if using English spearmint.

Medicinal – Spearmint tea is refreshing to drink on a hot, humid day. Spearmint also helps to prevent bad breath and is included in many toothpastes; it is good for the gums and helps whiten teeth. Mint can prevent milk from curdling. Like peppermint, spearmint has properties that help to dispel flatulence and, according to one eminent herbalist, the volatile oil in spearmint stimulates the digestive system and assists in cleansing the intestines.

Peppermint is one of the most valuable medicinal herbs. The fresh or dried leaves may be infused to make a tonic tea and it has excellent digestive properties. It also helps to relieve congestion in any part of the body, whether it is a headache, a cold, or bronchitis. The oil from the leaves was used long ago by the Chinese and Japanese.

Pennyroyal, like its mint relatives, is used by herbalists to remedy flatulence and griping pains in the abdomen. It is given to children in small amounts to ease fevers in measles and whooping cough. It promotes menstruation and is said to cause abortions, which is why it would not be advisable to offer it to young women. Country people do not like it in their pastures, where it grows freely, because it sometimes causes spontaneous abortion in cows. It is advised that this herb should never be boiled.

Culpeper has the final word by saying "All Mints are astringent and great strengtheners of the stomach".

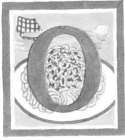

OREGANO
(O. vulgare) Labiatae
Perennial

Oregano has bright green, rather rough-textured foliage and is piercingly pungent. It grows in most aspects, with sun and well-drained soil being its main requirements. It reaches a height of 60 cm (2 ft) and has a spreading, though not invasive, root system. In summer and autumn the plant is frosted over with small white flowers (similar to those of marjoram) which are even more intense in flavour than the leaves. It is, in fact, one of the few herbs that are harvested while in bloom. The leaves and flowers are both used either fresh or dried, in cooking.

Propagation is by seed or cuttings in spring. Like marjoram, there are several varieties of oregano, some with smaller or larger leaves than *O. vulgare,* and the flowers can vary from light to dark pink in colour. All varieties of oregano have the same characteristic aroma and flavour. It is used extensively in Italian and Greek food, along with basil and garlic. The Greek name for oregano is *rigani.*

Oregano, being a member of the *labiatae* family, has many significant features. Dr. Rudolf Hauschka, in his deeply thought-provoking book "Nutrition" (still out of print as far as we know), says that all members of this plant group have a warming scent and taste. By merely rubbing, or chewing an oregano leaf, allowing the taste and smell to penetrate the senses, one begins to feel a glow of well-being, soothed and harmonized: these qualities, and more, are an aid to the metabolic forces. One of the distinguishing features of all *labiataes* is their rectangular stalks, and the leaves attached to them form a cross of opposing pairs when looked down on from above.

Uses:

Culinary – Oregano has a penetrating and hearty flavour. It is used extensively in the tasty regional dishes of many countries. It is a favourite herb for pasta and rice dishes, in pizzas, moussaka and tomato dishes. A pinch of oregano in an avocado dip adds relish. In everyday cooking, try it instead of thyme or mixed herbs in meatloaf and rissoles and on cooked, buttered zucchini (courgettes), capsicums (peppers) and eggplant (aubergines). Use it too to flavour beef, lamb, veal and pork.

Medicinal – Oregano has been a valued therapeutic herb in times past, and is still in use today by modern herbalists. It has much the same properties as marjoram, and in some cases is even more effective. It induces perspiration, eases griping pains and expels flatulence. An infusion of the herb is beneficial when taken at the onset of a fever, and it helps to soothe coughs.

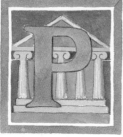

PARSLEY

(Petroselinum crispum) Umbelliferae
Biennial

There are varying opinions as to the regional origin of parsley, but it is generally thought to be Sardinia. It is a herb that has been known to mankind for centuries. Greek mythology says that it sprang from the blood of a Greek hero, Archemorous.

There are many different species of parsley; curled parsley includes sub-species called "triple-curled" and "moss-curled", their frilled green leaves being even more tightly crimped. The moss-curled variety makes an attractive border plant; it is low-growing and decorative as well as being useful. Italian parsley *(P. crispum neapolitanum)* is a much taller grow-ing, bushier type with flat, green leaves deeply indented at the edges. It is an excellent one to have growing in the garden because it is so good in soups and stews, the flavour being stronger than the curled varieties. Hamburg parsley *(P. sativum)* is yet another type but is not widely grown nowadays, although its long white root has culinary and medicinal uses.

Propagation for all types of parsley is by seed in spring. Autumn sowing is satisfactory where winters are mild. Grow the plants in a sunny position in average to rich, well-drained soil. The bed should be well watered, especially while the seeds are germinating, which can take up to two weeks. Although parsley is a biennial, it is

best to treat it as an annual and cut off the flower stalks as soon as they appear. The green umbels of flowers bloom in summer and their seeds are rich in an oil that is valuable in a medicinal substance called *apiol*. Once the plants have flowered they are spent and will wither.

In companion planting parsley is helpful to both roses and tomatoes, and bees visit the flowers constantly when they are in bloom.

Culpeper says parsley is under the dominion of Mercury and lists many ailments that are helped by the diffe-rent parts of the plant, which are pre-pared in various ways.

Uses:

Parsley is one of the most nutritious herbs, its roots, stems, leaves and seeds all having beneficial properties. The leaves, with their characteris-tically crisp texture, contain organic iron and vitamins, and the taste could be described as stimulating to the palate, with a mild, peppery bite and a pleasant earthy undertone. The flavour of parsley is not distinctively pungent, which makes it an excellent herb to use with others, giving "depth" to a blend. Parsley is one of the four used in *fines herbes,* the others being chervil, chives and tarragon in equal parts. It often goes into mixed herbs with thyme, sage and marjoram, and is traditional in a *bouquet garni,* together with a bay leaf and a sprig each of thyme and marjoram.

Chopped parsley leaves add flavour to mashed potatoes, omelettes, scrambled eggs, cream cheese, sauces (especially for fish), mornays, green salads, soups, pasta dishes and vegetable dishes. Parsley butter is good to eat with almost any grilled meats, or with baked jacket potatoes, and is easily made by beating the chopped leaves into softened butter, letting it harden on a plate in the refrigerator, then cutting it into rounds or squares. A quantity of chopped parsley incorporated into a scone mixture and then put on top of a simmering casserole, without the lid, and baked for about twenty minutes, is delicious. Parsley jelly is a pleasant accompaniment to meat, poultry and fish, and of course sprigs of parsley are invaluable as a garnish for almost any type of dish.

Medicinal – As parsley is rich in organic iron and other minerals it is helpful for anaemic conditions and also stimulates the appetite. It contains vitamims A, B and particularly vitamin C. Herbalists use a fluid extract from the roots to treat bladder, kidney and liver complaints. The oil from the seeds in carefully measured doses is used to treat menstrual problems. Parsley is a component in odourless garlic capsules. For domestic use, parsley leaves can be made into a tea which is helpful for bladder and kidney problems. Cooled parsley tea, or commercially prepared parsley lotion, closes enlarged pores and reduces puffiness around the eyes when dabbed on the face. It is also a good skin freshener. Chewing raw parsley is said to freshen the breath.

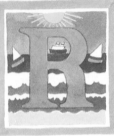

ROSEMARY

(*Rosmarinus officinalis*) Labiatae
Perennial

Rosemary evolved in the sun-drenched Mediterranean coastal regions where most of the pungent herbs we know so well had their beginnings. The Ancients held it in great esteem for many reasons: its remarkable healing qualities, its unique flavour, and for the mystical legends surrounding it, which led to its various symbolic meanings used in diverse ceremonies, even today. It is also a traditional symbol of remembrance.

Rosemary can be propagated by seeds, cuttings, or layering in spring (and in autumn in mild climates). It likes to grow in average to limy, well-drained soil in a sunny position, and thrives best near the sea. (Its Latin name means "dew of the sea".) When fully grown it reaches a height of 1.5 m (5 ft). It is covered in delicately coloured pale blue flowers which grow in clusters around the tips of the stems. They are filled with nectar and are a favourite with bees. Blooming starts in autumn and continues into spring and early summer, with occasional flowers appearing at other times. The erect, narrow leaves, with their fresh, resinous scent, abound in oil that is converted from sunlight and air by the plant's special chemistry. Commercially, the oil distilled from the flowering tops is finer than the oil from the leaves and stems.

There are other varieties of rosemary, some of which are widely grown and freely available, like the prostrate or horizontal rosemary (*R. officinalis prostratus*) which has smaller, more flexible foliage on long, curved branches which hang gracefully over walls during a long flowering period when the plant is massed with sky-blue blossoms. The more rare kinds of rosemary include a white flowering variety, another with a silver variegated leaf, one with a golden variegated leaf, and a pink flowering type. Another, more recent addition to our garden, has brilliant blue flowers of a deeper shade than any other we have seen. Locally it has the name of "Blue Lagoon", but it is also known as "Severn Sea" or "Benenden Blue". We saw it blooming freely and fragrantly at Sissinghurst Castle in Kent, and at Barbizon in France. Descriptions of these rare rosemarys are given by Guy Cooper and Gordon Taylor in their informative book *The Romance of Rosemary*, published by the British Herb Society in conjunction with The Juniper Press. Our "Blue Lagoon" has given us great pleasure, the prolific flowers smothering the bush for nine months of the year. The plant itself is neither upright or prostrate; it sends up several straight branches which then turn downwards in a flowing manner. It grows quite tall, however, in spite of its horizontal tendencies, and is approximately half the height of upright rosemary.

In astrology, Culpeper says "The Sun claims dominion over it."

Uses:

Culinary – Rosemary has a strong and distinctive flavour and helps to digest rich and starchy foods. It is important to cut the leaves very small, whether fresh or dried, because they are long and quite sharp and may be difficult to swallow otherwise. Rosemary is widely used in Greek and Italian cooking, often together with garlic. Cook rosemary with lamb, veal, pork, beef, rabbit and poultry to give the meat a delicious fragrance. It may be added to a liver pâté, and used in pasta dishes. Sprinkle some finely chopped leaves over buttered, cooked eggplant (aubergine), zucchini (courgette), Brussels sprouts and cabbage. It is very good in herb bread, and in a plain scone mixture, which sounds unusual but is quite delicious when eaten hot and generously buttered.

Medicinal – Rosemary is a healing herb and can be used to treat different parts of the body. It has been accepted for thousands of years that it helps all functions of the head, even the memory, hence the old saying "rosemary for remembrance". Greek students in the old days would twine sprigs of rosemary in their hair before studying, and herbalists today give tea of rosemary to strengthen the memory, to relieve headaches, to tone up the nervous system, to help the digestion, and to relieve colic. It is also reputed to strengthen the eyesight. Rosemary sprigs, or oil of rosemary, added to bath water is bracing and invigorating. It is especially good in the evening, to renew one's energy, before going out again at night. Do not have a rosemary bath just before going to bed, lavender is the herb to use as a sedative and calming bath at this time, as it soothes all the peripheral nerve endings of the body.

One of rosemary's best known therapeutic qualities is for the hair and scalp. Herbal shampoos and hair tonics that contain rosemary will revitalise the scalp, prevent (and cure) dandruff, and encourage the growth of new healthy hair. A rosemary hair rinse is easily made at home by simmering six to eight rosemary sprigs in a litre of water, with the lid on the saucepan, for ten to twenty minutes. Allow it to cool, then use it to rub into the hair and scalp during the final rinse.

Rosemary is also one of the components in eau-de-Cologne, and the dried flowers and leaves make a fragrant addition to a potpourri.

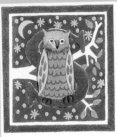

SAGE

(Salvia officinalis) Labiatae
Perennial

Garden sage originated from the sunny coasts of southern Europe. A combination of the special soil and climate must have been in harmonious collaboration to produce the numerous pungent herbs that are native to Mediterranean lands. Countless myths and legends surround many of these herbs and their divine source is attributed to Greek gods. A visitor to our garden, originally from Greece, was suddenly homesick when he saw and smelt the herbs and said that in his youth, wherever he walked, there was the powerful scent of crushed herbs underfoot. The scent was with him still, and he said that he had never encountered the strength of the perfume anywhere else.

According to one writer, there are more than 750 species of sage distributed throughout the world. The most important is *Salvia officinalis,* or garden sage, which has been cultivated for thousands of years for its medicinal and nutritional properties. The latin word *salvere,* from which the botanical title is derived, means "good health". The wholesome fragrance of sage leaves has a dry, pungent, yet lightly honeyed, undertone, giving an astringent relish to the palate when the leaves are nibbled. The grainy-looking, many-veined leaves are grey-green, and when growing in a clump with the dew still on them, the massed foliage has a nacreous luminosity. In early summer to autumn the violet-lipped flower cups are filled with nectar, which, according to Sir John Hill, M.D., an eighteenth century author, is "highly flavoured, balmy, fragrant resin, delicate to the taste, one of the most delicious cordials that can be thought of, warm and aromatic." Sage flowers are a great favourite with bees.

Propagation is by seeds or cuttings in spring (and in autumn in mild climates). Grow the plants in a sunny, elevated position in light to limy, well-drained soil. Sage plants grow to approximately 90 cm (3 ft).

Sage was introduced to Britain by the Romans, who also took it to the other countries where they settled. Great and varied application has been made of sage. It is used in wine, tea, cream, cheese, bread and tobacco, to name just a few of the uses to which this excellent herb has been put.

In companion planting, sage and rosemary grow well together, and cabbages are healthier when sage is grown amongst them.

Culpeper of course is full of praise for it, and says "Jupiter claims it". He also says "The juice taken in warm water, helps hoarseness and cough. Drank with vinegar, it is good for the plague."

Uses:

Culinary – Sage is a classic ingredient

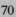

in mixed herbs, together with thyme and marjoram. It features in Mrs Beeton's famous recipe for Sage and Onion Stuffing for Roast Goose and Duck. Sage cuts the richness of certain foods, at the same time aiding in their digestion, which is why it complements pork, goose, duck, veal and oily fish. It also goes well with rich dairy foods and is a tasty addition to pea and bean soups. Add sage also to vegetable dishes featuring onions, eggplant (aubergines) or capsicums. Sage is good in cheese dishes, especially Welsh rarebit, some egg dishes, and gives a delicious aroma and flavour to dumplings and home-made bread.

Medicinal – A very old proverb says: "Why should a man die who has sage in his garden?" It was believed that sage helped to retard old age, prevent the loss of memory, and to give energy. It is known that sage was used by the ancient Egyptians as a brain tonic, and the Chinese believed that it promoted longevity, strengthed the memory and sharpened the senses. Sage tea is still taken today for its tonic effect on the liver, brain and nerves. An esteemed German homeopathic doctor told us that it helped all functions of the mouth and throat, and this was also known by the Ancients. It is still prescribed by practitioners of natural medicine as an excellent remedy for laryngitis and sore throats, when it is used as a gargle, or as a mouth wash for bleeding gums. It may be prepared for gargles or mouth washes by simmering two teaspoons of the freshly chopped leaves (or one teaspoon of the dried leaves) in one cup of milk (or water) in a saucepan, with the lid on, for several minutes. Strain through a fine sieve, pressing out the remaining sage leaf juices; cool and use. One herbalist suggests cider vinegar in place of the water or milk. Sage leaves rubbed over the gums and teeth is an old remedy for strengthening the gums and whitening the teeth. Some herbal toothpastes are made with sage as the main ingredient.

Sage was also used to restore the colour to greying hair. This was borne out when, after one of our lectures one day, a lady told us a fascinating story of the time when her grandmother worked as a cook in an English household. Apparently the butler was worried about losing his job because his hair was turning grey, so he would occasionally take a bunch of sage leaves to the cook and direct her to chop them finely and simmer them in some water until the liquid was reduced and thick with stewed sage. He would then comb this pomade through his hair, thereby darkening it, and assuring him of his position in the household!

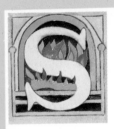

SAVORY

(Satureia montana) Labiatae
Perennial

Winter savory and its many relatives, including hyssop *(Hyssopus officinalis)*, also a Labiatae and used in the same way as savory), is native to the lands of the Mediterranean, and much of its history is shrouded in the mists of time. The Greeks and Romans knew its worth and introduced it to Britain. It was highly regarded for its pungent, warm scent and its value in nutrition and healing. Being typical of its generic family, "it is as though the whole plant had been dipped in aromatic fire forces from root to blossom, flooding one with a warm feeling of well-being", and enlivening the metabolic forces, as expressed so vividly by Rudolf Hauschka, D.Sc., in his book, *Nutrition.*

There are three kinds of savory most easily available and best known. Summer savory *(S. hortensis)* is an annual, growing to 60 cm (2 ft) with pink, summer-flowering blooms, soft stalks and stems, and tender leaves which are pepper-hot in flavour. Prostrate winter savory *(S. repandens)* is an ornamental perennial, blanketed in a snowdrift of white flowers in autumn, which are enticing to bees. It too has peppery, aromatic foliage, but stripping the leaves from the curving, ground-hugging stalks is a tedious task.

Winter savory, a perennial, is a bushy plant growing to 30 cm (12 inches), with pearly white blossoms from summer to autumn; these diminutive goblets are filled with nectar which bees find enchanting. The narrow, glossy green leaves are so sharply hot that if chewed for a few minutes, both tongue and palate object strongly! Winter savory puts out new soft growth in spring and summer, and this is when it is most pleasant to eat: in winter it becomes dwarfish, and the leaves change into hard little spikes that need to be chopped well and softened in liquid before using them. It takes a little experience when growing herbs to tell the difference between winter savory and garden thyme. Although they appear similar at first glance, their taste and scent are completely different.

Perennial winter and prostrate savories are propagated by seed, root division, or cuttings in spring (and in autumn in temperate climates). Summer savory is propagated by sowing seed in spring. Grow all savories in well-drained soil in a sunny position.

In Tudor England, winter savory was popular grown as a low hedge; the plants were set close together so that they grew into one another. The low, small-leaved box plant *(Buxus sempervirens)* was grown in the same way. Both need clipping for a typically neat appearance, and are delightful when used to outline the intricate patterns of "knot gardens", which are coming back into favour.

In the garden it associates well with beans, and is an insect repellent. Culpeper says it is a herb "under Mercury".

Uses:

Culinary – Savory is traditionally used with all kinds of beans, either fresh or dried, earning it the German name of *bohnen-kraut* and the Dutch *boonen kruid,* both meaning bean herb. Pepper herb is another popular name for savory. Beans and savory have long been a nutritional combination, not only for flavour, but also for digestion and health, as well as for deeper philosophical and spiritual reasons, which are explained fully in Rudolf Hauschka's *Nutrition*. This book makes fascinating reading for those who are interested in herbs.

Either summer and winter savory are both used and may be chopped and scattered over the beans when cooked, stirring in a little butter as well. Bean or lentil soups, too, are more aromatic and tasty when savory is added. There are other favourite ways of including it with beans, depending on the recipe and the type of bean.

Crumbled, dried savory, or fresh, chopped savory gives a zesty tang to breadcrumbs for coating fish, poultry, or other suitable meats before frying. If making your own sausages, or meat pies, savory makes an excellent and wholesome flavouring. An important fact for many people is that it may be used instead of pepper. It makes an excellent flavouring for herb vinegar and may be used with discretion in *fines herbes* for omelettes and salads.

Medicinal – Both summer and winter savory aid the digestion, the nervous system and the respiratory organs. Modern herbalists use savory as an intestinal antiseptic. Prepared as a tea, savory is still used to treat dyspepsia. One writer says that savory possesses aphrodisiac qualities. A well-known folk remedy for bee stings is to rub the spot with fresh savory leaves after removing the sting. Sprigs of savory added to bath water will tone and refresh the skin, or, alternatively, the fresh or dried savory can be put into a cheesecloth bag and infused in the hot water.

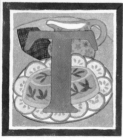

TARRAGON
(*Artemisia dracunculus*) Compositae
Perennial

Spicy French tarragon is native to the Mediterranean regions and has much more flavour than its relative, Russian tarragon, a native of Siberia. At first glance the two bear a resemblance to one other but on closer inspection it can be seen that French tarragon has straight, smooth, narrow leaves on wiry stems and does not look as lush or as green, and that Russian tarragon has indentations in its leaves and grows more prolifically. Russian tarragon has a very mild flavour and lacks the keen piquancy and warm aftertaste of French tarragon. In nutrition and medicine, French tarragon is true to the Compositae family, to which it belongs (wormwood is another member), carrying within its composition energies that are transformed by the plant from various natural sources, giving it individual aroma and beneficial properties. In mythology, plants belonging to the genus *Artemisia* were dedicated to Artemisia, Goddess of Nature and twin sister of Apollo.

If for any reason you cannot obtain or grow French tarragon, an excellent substitute is winter tarragon, *Tagetes lucida*. Its flavour is more pungent, forceful, and less subtle, and its leaves are coarser and rougher, but it is widely used in areas where French tarragon is difficult to grow.

French tarragon grows in a tangle of stems and leaves and produces in summer tiny bud-like "flowers" which do not mature and bear seed, although the plant has been known to do so in parts of France. It grows to 90 cm (3 ft) and is reproduced by cuttings or root division in late spring. It grows best in light, well-drained soil, and must be watered well in dry weather or the leaves will soon wilt. During the coldest part of winter the foliage withers, yellows, and dies, although the serpentine root system is hibernating underground and will send up new green shoots in spring. Mark the spot with a coloured stake so that the dormant root is not dug up by mistake, and spread a little mulch over the root area to help keep out the cold, and if the weather is dry, water well from time to time.

In companion planting, this aromatic herb is beneficial generally to the rest of the garden. Culpeper says it is "a mild martial plant", and that the leaves are "heating and drying", a fact that modern herbalists are aware of.

Uses:

Culinary – French tarragon is unique in its seductive flavour and cannot be substituted in certain dishes that call for its inclusion (with the possible exception of a small amount of winter tarragon). It is one of the subtle, yet distinctive herbs that make up a *fines herbes* blend (in equal quantities with parsley, chives and chervil, all chopped finely), and it has become traditional to set a few leaves in a delicate chilled salmon *en gelée,* a summer treat that is served with finely sliced cucumber and Hollandaise sauce. The leaves lend themselves admirably for setting in moulds and terrines, both for appearance and flavour, and can be arranged to form attractive patterns.

French tarragon is an essential ingredient of Béarnaise sauce, helping to give it its distinctive taste, and into Tartare sauce. The finely chopped leaves are excellent when folded into mayonnaise, melted butter sauce, sour cream dressing and French dressing. It also makes a delicious herb butter: mash the finely chopped leaves into softened butter, add a squeeze of lemon, spread on a plate and leave to set in the refrigerator. To use, cut it into circles or cubes and place on top of cooked fish, steak, or cutlets. Delicate meat, such as chicken, shellfish and fish, benefit from the tart aroma of tarragon, and it goes equally well in egg dishes, mornays, and with veal, liver or kidneys, and in vegetable or fish soups.

Tarragon vinegar, used in French dressing, is perennially popular and is made by putting quantities of fresh tarragon sprays in a jar and filling it to the top with white wine vinegar and replacing the lid. Infuse on a sunny window sill for two weeks and decant into a clean bottle. A few fresh sprays can be added to the decanted vinegar before sealing the bottle. Chopped tarragon in mustard gives it a special flavour, and it is often added to French mustard.

Medicinal – French tarragon leaves contain an essential volatile oil. French tarragon is reputed to stimulate the appetite and assist digestion, and, because of its diuretic properties, helps to rid the body of excess fluids. Herbalists today prescribe an infusion of the leaves to relieve flatulence. The root of tarragon was once used to ease the discomfort of toothache.

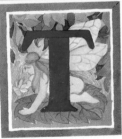

THYME

(*Thymus vulgaris*) Labiatae
Perennial

Most writers of Herbals, spanning several hundred years, agree that thyme is possibly the oldest herb known to man. It is believed to be native to the Mediterranean region, where it has the strongest perfume, and has become naturalised in many other countries through the centuries. Some botanists maintain that thyme leaves are one of the most primitive in form, never having developed into a more complex shape: each tiny, perfectly plain, oval leaf is attached by a minute stem to stiff, branching stalks in serried rows. The flowers, although many-hued, according to their variety, are identical in shape. The main flower head is a mass of minuscule blossoms grouped close together in circlets at the top of the plant. The bush types have flowers at intervals down the leaf stalks as well.

There are many varieties of this well-known herb, including carpeting and creeping thymes with white, crimson, pink, or mauve flowers, and other decorative ones with silver, or gold, streaked foliage, velvet-soft, grey, woolly leaves, and bright lime-green leaves. Garden thyme (a cultivated form of wild thyme), lemon thyme, and Westmoreland thyme are three varieties that are upright and bushy, and

are more than merely ornamental. Garden thyme has an intensely pungent aroma and flavour and is the most valuable in food and medicine. When fully mature the leaves are a light grey; the plant grows to 30 cm (12 inches) and bears creamy-pink, spring-flowering blooms. Lemon thyme (*T. citriodorus*) is a lower, thicker plant than garden thyme, with glossy green foliage, lavender-coloured flowers in summer, and a distinct and delicous lemon scent. Westmoreland thyme is akin to garden thyme in perfume and taste, although less intense. It is a lower, spreading plant with densely packed leaves of dusky green, and in spring is cloaked in rosy blossoms that provide a fragrant, honeyed feast for bees.

Legends recount that thyme has always been a favourite fairy herb, and one cannot help thinking of Ariel in Shakespeare's *The Tempest* when he says: "Where the bees suck, there suck I." Thyme honey has a particularly delicate aroma, and when it comes from Mount Hymettus in Greece, it is the most prized of all. Tasting rare and exquisitely fragrant, fine-textured thyme honey from a small stone pot, one could easily imagine that it was indeed the food of fairies. Thyme absorbs sunlight, as well as special air and soil

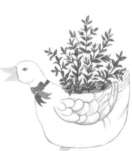

elements which it transforms into valuable substances and oils, becoming refined essences in the leaves and flowers, especially strong in garden thyme, the variety highly esteemed both in herbal medicine and therapeutic products.

All varieties of thyme are perennial and are propagated by seed, cuttings, or root division in spring. They thrive in sandy soil in the sun, abhorring damp, shady places, where they are liable to wither and die. Gritty soil gives the creeping and spreading thymes something for the searching stems and rootlets to cling to; several varieties planted together in well-forked, limed soil with a judicious sprinkling of gravel, in a sunny area interspersed with stepping stones, makes a charming, perfumed nook for a thyme collection. If the different varieties grow into one another it does not matter, and a few mounding thymes, like *T. nitidus,* and some small, lichened boulders placed at intervals in the thyme sea, will all add to the pleasing, rather magical, appearance of the scene.

As well as being an essential culinary and medicinal herb, thyme is used in herbal toothpastes, mouth washes and in natural cosmetics. Put some fresh sprigs of thyme into a facial steam for toning up the skin.

In companion planting, thyme, as an exceptionally aromatic herb, has a livening effect on all plants and associates well with lavender. It helps to repel cabbage moths in the vegetable garden, and when dried and put into bags acts as a moth repellent when hung in cupboards and placed in drawers.

The herbalist-astrologer, Dr Culpeper, lists thyme as "a notable herb of Venus".

Uses:
Culinary – The pungent garden thyme is blended with sage and marjoram for mixed herbs and when doing this yourself it is simpler to use the dried herb, as fresh thyme leaves, being so small and tenacious, take a lot of patient stripping from the stalks if a large quantity is required. Whole sprays of fresh garden thyme, with marjoram, parsley and a bay leaf tied together with a long piece of string, go into making a *bouquet garni,* which is added to certain dishes that need to be cooked for a long time; remove the bunch by the long string at the end of the cooking time, when most of the leaves will have become almalgamated into the food. If using dried *bouquet garni,* add a teaspoon or two at the beginning of cooking time so that the herbs can become part of the savoury essences released by the other ingredients. Or, if the *bouquet garni* is contained in a sachet (sometimes called for in recipes where the dish has a clear, finished appearance, such as a hot or cold jellied consommé), remove it at the end of the cooking time.

Thyme may be used on its own if you prefer a stronger flavour, or temper it with parsley, marjoram, sage and chives. Either on its own or mixed with other herbs, it is indispensable in soups, stews and casseroles. Tasty sausages that some butchers used to make were flecked with thyme and other herbs, whereas nowadays, sadly, manufactured essences are mainly used. A thyme mixture gives flavour and nutritional value to meat loaves, rissoles, and other meat dishes. It is traditional in stuffings and marinades. Put a pinch in a pâté or a terrine. Thyme in herb bread gives an excellent, mouthwatering flavour. A few fresh (stalkless!) leaves sprinkled over cooked and buttered vegetables is another way of using fresh thyme on its own.

Westmoreland thyme, although several degrees milder, may be used in the same way as garden thyme. Lemon thyme, with its refreshing citrus overtones, is excellent when cooking fish, chicken and other white or delicate meats, or in mornays of turkey, chicken, or egg, as well as in omelettes and cheese soufflés. Some cooks maintain that a *fines herbes* blend is not complete without lemon thyme to go with the chervil, tarragon, parsley and chives.

Medicinal – Top grade thyme oil is distilled from the fresh leaves and flowering tops of garden thyme, which contains many constituents. Thymol (made from thyme oil) is a powerful antiseptic and is highly regarded for medicinal use, the French variety being considered the best. Commercially, thymol is sometimes mixed with other oils, and coloured with root substances but this is considered inferior to the pure oil.

Modern herbalists use thyme, prepared in various ways, to aid the digestion, to relieve flatulence and colic, and to remedy bowel disorders. Thyme also helps to cut phlegm and relieves throat and bronchial ailments. It improves the appetite, relieves headaches, acts as a nerve tonic, and "clears the brain". For a quick pick-me-up, try a cup of hot thyme tea, and hold the pungent herb to your nostrils as well. Thyme is also believed to improve the eyesight and has the reputation of toning up the reproductive system.

Culpeper declares in his *Herbal* that: "An ointment made of it takes away hot swellings and warts..." it is excellent for those troubled with gout:... and it eases pains in the loins and hips. Taken inwardly, the herb comforts the stomach and expels wind."

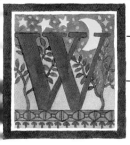

WATERCRESS

(Nasturtium officinale) Cruciferae
Perennial

There are a number of different types of cress – perennial watercress and a variety of annuals, all with the same, biting, peppery taste, and all are rich in natural iron. Propagation for watercress is either by seed or root division in spring, and autumn in temperate climates. Land, or garden, cress *(Lapidium sativum)* is propagated by seed in spring, and autumn too if conditions are mild in winter. All cresses like to grow in semi-shade, or in full shade, in loamy soil. Watercress will flourish in a damp spot in the garden, or in a container under a dripping tap; flood the container with water once a week and tip out the excess. Watercress should never grow in stagnant water; the ideal place is either in a running stream or on its banks, where the water will wash over the roots of the plants. Watercress grows to a height of 45 cm (1 ½ ft) while land cress is about 15 cm (6 inches) high, or smaller.

Watercress originally came from Europe and parts of Asia, while history says land cress is native to Persia. Both watercress and land cress (as well as mustard) belong to the Cruciferae family, so called because the four petals of the flowers of each of these plants – whatever their size or colour – form a Greek cross. There are no poisonous plants among the two thousand species of this genus. The garden nasturtium *(Tropaelum majus),* sometimes called Indian cress, is not classed as one of the cresses mentioned here because of some botanical differences, but it too belongs to the Cruciferae family; its leaves and flowers are high in vitamin C and may be eaten in salads and sandwiches.

Watercress has a creeping habit and sends out long, sappy stems along the ground with masses of rootlets attached. Stems and leaves also shoot up from the plant and these are the ones to gather. In summer the plant is frosted over with tiny white flowers which should be cut off from the base of their stems to keep the plant growing vigorously.

Land cress remains as one single plant, and among the varieties is "mustard-cress" which can be bought in punnets and which crop only once: when the little leaves are cut the plant stops growing. Another variety, French cress, looks like a miniature clump of lettuce, with fine-textured, broadish leaves, frilled at the edges. This too will not continue to grow once the leaves are picked. Similarly, curled cress, which looks like a fleshy parsley. The most rewarding land cress to grow is the American upland cress which grows in a layered rosette of indented leaves rather like a dandelion in shape. It will grow for a year and the leaves can be picked frequently from the outside, allowing new growth from the centre.

Upland cress sends up long stems bearing yellow flowers in spring, which is the time to pull it out and start again.

Culpeper says watercress is under the dominion of the Moon, and also advises that "The leaves bruised, or the juice, is good to be applied to the face or other parts troubled with freckles, pimples, spots, or the like, at night, and washed away in the morning".

Uses:

Culinary – Cress of any kind is so nutritious that it should be used unstintingly. Be lavish with cress in green salads: tear up whole leaves or chop them up finely. The foliage is always attractive used as a garnish. Cress sandwiches are very popular: chop any of the cresses finely, and lay them thickly on thin brown or white buttered bread, cover with more buttered bread, remove the crusts and cut into fingers or triangles – perfect for afternoon tea, or as an accompaniment to soups and entrées. Cress soup is a green and delectable start to a meal and can be served piping hot in winter or icy cold in summer.

Medicinal – Watercress is particularly rich in organic iron, and naturopaths advocate its use, especially for those who cannot assimilate iron tablets. Watercress is also rich in vitamins and minerals and contains sulphur, iodine and phosphorus. It is a natural blood purifier and is said to clear the complexion, brighten the eyes, and remove disfiguring blackheads and pimples, if used continuously.

"Watercress pottage [soup] is a good remedy to cleanse the blood in the spring, and helps head-aches, and consumes the gross humours winter hath left behind" sayeth Dr Culpeper!

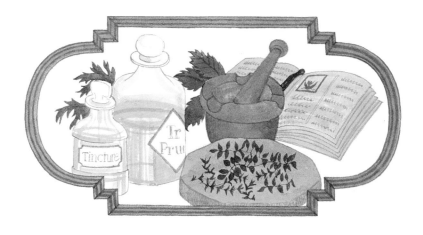

HERBS
AS
MEDICINE

The benefits of orthodox (allopathic) medicine have long been recognised and the advances in scientific research and modern technology have often brought dramatic and life-saving discoveries. In spite of this, alternative forms of healing and prevention of illness are becoming more widely recognised and accepted. One of the reasons for this may be that people are becoming more aware of the side effects of chemically manufactured drugs and are turning to more natural forms of healing, some of which are discussed briefly below.

Naturopathy is one form of alternative medicine. After diagnosis, the patient is advised on diet and inner cleansing and is treated with herbal medicines, tablets, ointments, teas and special oils. These treatments are sometimes used in conjunction with various therapeutic skills including massage, manipulation, acupuncture, colour therapy, and aromatherapy, the last an art practised by the ancient Egyptians which has been revived and pioneered in recent times by Margaret Maury. In aromatherapy, skilled practitioners prescribe certain oils, which, according to the ailment, may either be used internally, massaged into the skin, or used to purify the air. Physiotherapists who are trained in this therapy claim to be able to change a person's mood by using oils with different aromas – some oils are said to improve the memory, others help concentration and meditation, induce tranquillity, influence recovery from illness, and so on.

As with any form of healing, it is important to seek the advice of a registered, experienced and reputable practitioner since some forms of inner cleansing used in naturopathy are no longer considered advisable.

Homoeopathy, another form of healing, is very highly regarded and has also the Royal seal of approval. In the 18th century Dr Samuel Hahnemann, a German physician, after long observation, successful treatment of patients, and study, revealed this particular form of medicine. "Like cures like" is one of the basic principles of homoeopathy. Medicines are made from plants, trees, flowers, weeds, minerals, and some animal products. They are individually prepared so that they may be given to patients in small, diminishing doses, until the 'trilogy' of mind, body, and spirit are activated to partake in the healing process. People on homoeopathic treatment keep a range of these medicines, which they use every day, and even have a special kit to use when travelling.

Bach Remedies, discovered by Dr Edward Bach in the 1930s, also have a distinguished reputation; they are made from the essential energy found within flowers and trees. The essences are extracted in a unique way and are meticulously prepared for individual use, in a way that is similar to homoeopathy.

There are a great many specialist homoeopathic doctors throughout the world today, many of whom have also completed their orthodox medical training, and who prescribe homoeopathic and Bach Remedies for their patients.

The remedies and cures detailed in this chapter are merely household 'simples' and are not intended to replace any medication that may have been prescribed by a doctor or other registered practitioner. Some of these household remedies have been quoted from *Lotions and Potions* and some are from Dr Künzle's *Herbs and Weeds*. Naturopathy, homoeopathy, and Bach Remedies require study, training, and a thorough background

knowledge, which take many years to acquire.

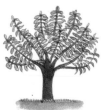

Some old and well-tried home remedies

Many years ago, when we first decided to make the growing and processing of herbs our livelihood and way of life, a very kind English aunt, the late Mrs Thomas Dodd, sent us a most enchanting little book called *Lotions and Potions,* which was a collection of "Recipes of Women's Institute Members and their Ancestors", edited by Gwynedd Lloyd and printed in England by Novello and Co. Ltd, in 1956. This delightful book, with its cheerful blue and yellow cover depicting a country cottage surrounded by flowers, a many-paned window left invitingly open, birds perching on the sloping, thatched roof, and pet cats on the path, has been a great source of interest and knowledge, and a number of the household remedies within its pages have been quoted, and acknowledged, in books we have written. It is still treasured amongst our reference books, and is now showing signs of all the thumbing and reading it has had through the years.

Imagine our delight when, visiting Culpeper's fascinating and charming shop in Cambridge recently, we saw a new edition of this book on their shelves, printed by Bournemouth Press Ltd, Bournemouth – this time with an evocative musk-pink cover. Naturally we bought it immediately. We should like to borrow a few more of the common-sense and useful recipes from a favourite book.

From Lotions and Potions:

A lotion for baldness

"Take of box leaves four handfuls. Boil in eight pints of water in a tightly closed pan for fifteen minutes. Add an ounce of Eau-de-Cologne. Wash the head every evening."

N.B. Box leaves come from *Buxus sempervirens.*

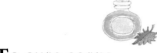

To cure corns

"Wash the feet in hot salted water. Squeeze a drop of the juice of the greater Celandine *(Chelidonium majus)* onto the corn and leave to dry. Two applications are usually sufficient. This cure can also be used for warts."

N.B. The book attributes this cure to an "old herbal".

Bruise oil

"Balm, rosemary, chamomile flowers, rosebuds, feverfews, sage, lavender tops, southernwood betony, wormwood.

Take of each a handful and chop them small, put in a stone jar with sufficient salad oil to cover them. Stand for a fortnight, stirring often. Then boil gently till the oil is extracted (till ingredients become crisp), but do not exceed the heat of boiling water. Strain through linen, and keep in well-corked bottle. A well-tried receipt."

Infusion for nervous headaches and bad memory

"One ounce fresh or dried rosemary, infused with one pint of boiling water. Cool and strain.

Dose: a wineglassful 4 times a day – hot."

Rheumatism

"Boil 1 oz of celery seed in 1 pint of water until reduced to half. Strain, bottle and cork carefully. Take 1 teaspoonful twice a day in a little water for a fortnight. Repeat again if required."

Chilblain mixture

"Mix one tablespoonful of honey with equal quantity of glycerine, the white of an egg and enough flour to make a paste – a teaspoonful of rosewater may be added. Wash the affected parts with warm water, dry and spread on paste. Cover with piece of linen or cotton material."

So many people have been sincerely interested and generous to us during the long years of our rewarding "herbal experience". One person in particular, whom we have never met, has a special place in our thoughts. He is the gentleman who sent us a dear and quaint little book, full of wisdom and sound advice, called *Herbs and Weeds,* by "Father John Künzle, Herbalist." The new copy we have been able to find was printed by Salvioni and Co. SA., Bellinzona, Switzerland, in 1975.

John Künzle was born in Switzerland in 1857. He wished to devote himself to God's service and was ordained after graduating from the seminary of St. Gall. He then, through various circumstances, continued studying botany, a favourite subject, and soon became aware of the healing powers of herbs. After many case histories, and a rigorous examination by a board of physicians, which he passed brilliantly, he was acknowledged by the authorities as a Father-herbalist and became world famous. He was able to understand man in his entirety, taking into account the interaction of body and soul; he also had an intuitive flair for the hidden healing powers of herbs and was a pioneer in the science of poisonless herb healing. His booklet *Herbs and Weeds,* edited in 1911, was published in German and has been translated into several languages.

In 1945, at the age of 87, Father Künzle died of a heart attack, "but still in rare mental vigour... he passed to the better world, to the blessed Kingdom where the most beautiful alpine flowers and the finest herbs will flourish and smell sweet for him".

From *Herbs and Weeds.*

A simple remedy for corns

Many people cut onions in slices, lay them in vinegar and place a slice on the corn every night. It helps many. But usually vanity is to be blamed for all these corns because people wear too small shoes.

Influenza tea

To prevent influenza, drink a sip of a tea prepared from the following mixture in the morning and evening: one handful each of wormwood, sage, Alpine speedwell, and liquorice root. People who are sick with influenza should take a spoonful of this tea every half-hour. They will recover in two days.

Orange blossoms – *Flores aurantil*

Orange blossoms are considered to be a very pleasant and absolutely harmless sedative for the nerves which explains why they are mainly used as an ingredient for teas to calm the nerves and to encourage sleep. They are also suitable for correcting the scent and taste in remedies.

Wild pansy – *Herba violae tricoloris*

Wild pansy blossoms are a blood-purifying remedy in case of skin diseases (eczema, milk-crust, acne, furunculosis). They stimulate both urination and metabolism and are therefore used for stomach and bladder troubles, weakness of the kidneys, micturition, gravel, articular rheumatism, gout, and arteriosclerosis; also in case of heart disturbances, hysteria, chronic bronchial catarrh, and cramps.

N.B. This pretty little wild pansy, an annual, is often known as heartsease, Johnny-jump-up, and love-in-idleness.

Some simple home remedies and hints

● For simple household burns, caused by touching a hot iron in the wrong place, or grasping an overheated saucepan handle, and the like, gently pat lavender oil over the sore part. This will not only take away the pain, but will help to heal the skintissue.

● For a sweet-smelling bathroom, pour a few drops of a flower oil on to the spout of the hot tap and turn it on for a few moments to release the fragrance. The floral aroma will fill the room for some time.

● During a flea plague, fresh pennyroyal sprigs, or oil of pennyroyal, should be rubbed into the coats of dogs and cats. If fleas invade the house, put sprigs of pennyroyal wherever you can, even under mattresses. If you do not have fresh pennyroyal, use pennyroyal oil, which is even more concentrated.

• Insect bites are alleviated by rubbing the skin with fresh sage leaves. The pain of a bee-sting is lessened if the area is rubbed with fresh leaves of winter or summer savory – after first removing the sting.

• Lavender oil rubbed into some of the furniture, or bunches of fresh lavender in vases, helps to keep houseflies at bay. A posy of rue, tansy, wormwood and elder leaves is excellent for this purpose too.

• Chewing strawberries will prevent the formation of tartar on your teeth.

• Cinnamon bark pieces, dried wormwood leaves and the dried leaves of tansy and mint crumbled together and put into muslin bags will help keep moths and silverfish away from cupboards and drawers.

• For restless legs syndrome, during the night, put your legs in a bath of hot water up to the calves and pour in a few drops of soothing lavender oil. Soak them for five minutes, rubbing gently with a washer. Dry your legs and go back to bed. It helps the condition, but does not cure it.

• Plant tansy near entrances to the house to prevent the small, black summer flies, who somehow find a way inside, in spite of fly-screens. (This has been proved effectively by us.) Tansy, together with rue, wormwood, laven-

der, and a small elder tree planted around a barbecue area has the same effect. Sprays of tansy placed on an outdoor buffet also help to repel flies. Unfortunately it is too bitter to eat.

• A strong wormwood tea, cooled, and poured on the tracks of slugs and snails in spring and autumn will deter them.

To lose weight

"For the normal healthy person who is falling into flesh the safest and best method of slimming to adopt is to eat much less of all food taken as a usual thing at meals. It is also necessary to refrain from eating between meals." From *The Coronation Cookery Book* compiled for the Country Women's Association of N.S.W., Australia, by Jessie Sawyer O.B.E. and Sara-Moore-Sims.

And from the same book:

A good eyewash

"One dram boracic powder, ½ oz witchhazel, 2 grains sulphate of zinc, 8 oz rose water.
  Dilute with two or three parts of warm water, and apply by means of eyebath."

A doctor's preventive for influenza

"Take 2 drops of oil of cinnamon on sugar daily."

For cleansing the digestive system

A herbal tea made from the fresh or dried leaves of lovage taken twice a day for one or two weeks. To be included in fresh green salads as well.

Date and fig cure

An excellent mild laxative, and one which children usually take to readily.

315 g (10 oz) dates
125 g (4 oz) figs

Wash the dried fruit, stone the dates, mix with the figs and either put them through the medium cutter of a mincer, or put into a blender and chop only until the mixture resembles breadcrumbs. Using your hands, form the mixture into a ball by holding it under running cold water and pressing and squashing until the fruit holds together. Place the ball on a clean surface and roll it into a long sausage shape. Cut into pieces about 2.5 cm (1 inch) long. Store in refrigerator.

A comfortable cordial to cheer the heart

"Take one ounce of conserve of gilliflowers, four grains of the best Musk bruised as fine as flour, then put into a little tin pot and keep it till you have need to make this Cordial following: Take the quantity of one nutmeg out of your tin pot, put to it one spoonful of Cinnamon-water, and one spoonful of the Sirup of Gilliflowers, Ambergris, mix all these together, and drink them in the morning, fasting three or four hours, this is most comfortable." "A Choice Manual of Secrets in Physick", Elizabeth Grey, Countess of Kent, 1653, in A Garden of Herbs, Eleanour Sinclair Rohde, published for the Medici Society Ltd, London, by Philip Lee Warner.

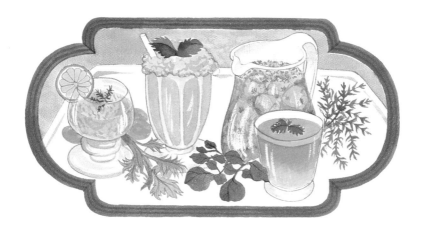

HERB TEAS
AND
BEVERAGES

A tea or "coffee" made from the leaves, flowers, bark, seeds, berries, or roots of certain herbs makes a pleasing, healthful drink for those who prefer a change from conventional tea and coffee. These beverages may be taken at any time of the day – first thing in the morning, at mid-morning, at lunch time, in the afternoon, after dinner, and before going to bed. They can be taken either hot or iced. Each one has different benefits and can assist in overcoming mild or chronic indispositions. As a preventive measure, taking specific herb teas over a period of time builds up a resistance to a number of illnesses. Herbs are potent in their own way, and their use should be balanced.

Herb teas are becoming increasingly popular and are being accepted by people in parts of the world other than the continental and Asian countries where they have always been popular. An improvement in health can often be noticed after having taken various kinds; it is also interesting to notice how clean one's palate feels after drinking a herb tea. Some teas are instantly enjoyed, most are pleasant to drink, others may take a little longer to gain favour and should be mixed with another well-liked herb, or a natural flavouring, to make them more palatable.

A herbal tea is an infusion of boiling water and herbs, either fresh or dried. The leaves are the most effective in some cases, and the seeds, berries, bark, flowers or roots in others. Keep a separate teapot for these teas, and when using the dried leaves, powdered root, crushed seeds or berries, put one teaspoon for each cup into the pot and pour boiling water onto them; allow to infuse for about three minutes, then strain into cups. If using fresh herb leaves for tea, use twice the quantity than the dried, and infuse for several minutes longer. For flower teas, either fresh or dried, use the same amount as you would for the leaves. The traditional method for flower teas, to extract the most from them, is to bring a small saucepan (not aluminium) of measured water to the boil, add the flowers, put the lid on and simmer for one minute. Allow the tea to stand for a little longer, then strain into cups.

A number of herb teas of various kinds are now available, either on their own or as a blend in teabags, and are gaining in esteem. The bags are infused in the usual way, by pouring freshly boiled water over them.

A tea worth mentioning is made from the valerian plant, *Valeriana officinalis,* the most beneficial part being the root, which is dried and ground. If growing your own, when the plant is mature dig out the root, wash it, cut into slices and allow to dry until dehydrated. Grind to a powder, or into small granules, in the blender. The common dandelion, *Taraxacum officinale,* is another plant whose root makes a beneficial beverage. The fresh leaves are also of great value to eat. Dandelion root can be bought already ground, or granulated, and for some reason is not called dandelion tea, but "coffee" or "beverage". Root teas are made in the same way as leaf teas. A bark beverage that is extremely therapeutic is slippery elm bark tea, and is made quite differently from any teas we have mentioned (see page 93).

Two teas may be mixed, especially if the flowers are complementary and they do not both give the same benefits. In this way the value of the tea may be doubled. A litre may be made at the beginning of the day and stored in the refrigerator.

No milk is added to herb teas.

Honey, a squeeze of lemon, orange-flower water or rose water (the last two are usually available from continental or Greek delicatessens) can be stirred into the tea if you wish. In the summer, ice cubes, long stalks of fresh, leafy herbs and a little mineral water or fresh fruit juice, all help to enhance the taste of these teas.

Many herb teas, or infusions as they are often called, are excellent lotions for the skin, giving it a natural, soft bloom. The infusion must be cooled first, then lightly patted on to the face and neck with soaked balls of cotton wool.

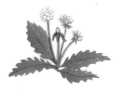

Angelica leaf or root tea
All parts of angelica are health-giving. A tea made from the fresh or dried leaves is excellent for colds or influenza, and for soothing the nerves. The bruised root made into a tea relieves flatulence. The pleasant flavour of the leaves makes it suitable to mix with other herb teas which do not have such a pleasing taste. Pour angelica leaf tea into a hot bath for relaxation and fragrance.

Aniseed tea
This tea is made from the seeds, which should be crushed to release the medicinal oils. Allow this tea to draw for a little longer. It relieves indigestion and flatulence, is helpful in allaying colds, and brightens the eyes. It also freshens the palate and sweetens the breath. Small amounts of aniseed, ground to a powder, may be added to the food of young children to help their digestion. A warm milk and honey beverage with a little powdered aniseed added

will help to soothe a fretful child. It is strongly advised that these simple home remedies should be given in moderation to very young children, and as they grow older the strength can be increased gradually. Moisten cotton wool pads in cooled aniseed tea and apply to the skin to lighten it.

Balm leaf tea
Lemon balm tea helps to reduce high temperatures as it induces perspiration. It also lessens the effects of exhaustion in hot weather. This tea assists the digestion and the appetite, helps to settle an upset stomach and eases griping pains in the stomach. It is also an anti-depressant. Double strength balm tea in a hot bath cleanses and perfumes the skin.

Basil leaf tea
A tea of basil leaves is good for the lungs and diseases of the kidneys and bladder. Basil leaves infused in wine and patted on to the face helps to close enlarged pores. It combines well with borage leaf tea.

Bay leaf tea
A tea of bay leaves is excellent for the digestion and is somewhat astringent as well. A facial steam bath, for cleansing and clearing the skin, is made in the same way as the tea, with the addition of chamomile flowers, rosemary leaves and rose petals (all either fresh or dried). This was a popular beauty treatment in days of old.

Bergamot leaf tea
A tea made from this herb was favoured by the American pioneers as a remedy for sore throats and chest complaints; it was a cure they learned from the Indians. The tea poured into a hot bath is revitalising and perfumes the water delightfully.

Borage leaf tea
A tea of borage is used as a heart tonic, as a stimulant for the adrenal glands, and as a purifier to the system. It was once said to engender courage and to give confidence to the timid. Mixed with basil it assists the kidneys and bladder, heart and glands, as well as generally strengthening the system. Used as a facial steam, a tea made from the leaves and flowers of borage improves dry, sensitive skin.

Caraway seed tea
This tea is made in the same way as aniseed tea and it has many of the same benefits. Crush the seeds slightly before pouring on the boiling water. It is beneficial to the liver, gall bladder and digestion and eases the discomfort of flatulence. It assists the activity of the glands and increases the action of the kidneys. Owing to caraway's digestive and cleasing properties, it is helpful in clearing the complexion.

Carob bean tea
Tea made from carob comes from the dried bean of the small carob tree, *Ceratonia siliqua,* native to the Mediterranean coastal regions. It is also known as St. John's Bread. It is being widely used by manufacturers of health foods as an excellent substitute for chocolate and cocoa. Carob "confectionery" is a good alternative to sugar-based products and will help to prevent decay in children's teeth, as well as being more nutritious. Carob powder is also a corrective in cases of diarrhoea.

Chamomile flower tea
This is one of the best known herb teas. Make it in the way suggested for flower teas at the beginning of this chapter. Chamomile tea has long been used as a soothing beverage and is

especially helpful when taken before going to bed. Tea made from the flowers of German chamomile, an annual, is considered to have more potency than that made from perennial English chamomile; German chamomile also blooms more prolifically. For menstrual pain and nervous tension take a cup of chamomile tea. When the brain is overactive and tired, as when studying for exams, a cup of chamomile tea taken before going to bed, and after a hot bath with a few drops of lavender oil in it (lavender soothes the nerve endings of the body), will help to induce sound, natural sleep. A *very weak* chamomile tea sweetened with honey is helpful for young children who are overtired, or who are teething. Chamomile tea, double strength, is excellent in a herbal bath and will reduce fatigue; it can be used together with lavender oil. An infusion of chamomile flowers, when cooled, makes a brightening hair rinse, and if one has normally blond highlights, the chamomile will make it even fairer, especially if it is used over a long period of time.

Chervil leaf tea

Chervil has always been valued as a blood purifier and was considered an excellent tea to take in the spring. It helps the kidneys as well, and used to be taken to ease rheumatic conditions. Cloths soaked in the tea, wrung out, and applied to swellings and bruises, help to reduce them. It is said to purify the system and to brighten dull eyes and clear the complexion.

Chicory root tea or coffee

Chicory beverage is from the roots, which are roasted and ground and, like dandelion, is called "coffee". It is excellent when recovering from a bilious attack and hepatitis, and is generally good for the liver and gall bladder. It also has laxative prop-

erties, as well as helping to rid the body of excess fluids. However, it is not recommended for people who are anaemic. Sometimes chicory root is blended with real coffee.

Chive leaf tea

A tea made from chopped fresh chive leaves will stimulate the appetite, have a tonic effect on the kidneys, and is said to lower the blood pressure. As chives are a source of calcium, chive tea helps to strengthen nails and teeth.

Comfrey leaf tea

Comfrey tea has been a country remedy for countless ages and is used to heal internal injuries and broken bones, hence its common name of "knitbone". It contains a large amount of calcium and vitamin B12. Because of these properties it helps in the formation of strong teeth and bones. It also helps the circulation and cleanses the bloodstream. It is said to benefit those suffering from ulcers caused by varicose veins. Poultices soaked in strong comfrey tea can be applied to injured muscles and areas of bone weakness. The cooled tea patted on to the skin makes an excellent tonic for the complexion.

Coriander seed tea

Coriander, like other seed teas, is more powerful when the seeds are slightly crushed and the tea is left to infuse for longer than leaf teas. It too is excellent for the digestion, relieving griping pains and flatulence, especially after eating carbohydrates. It is another herb tea which has been used traditionally for purifying the blood, thus clearing the complexion.

Cress leaf tea

All cresses are rich in vitamins and minerals, especially watercress, and contain sulphur, iron, iodine and phosphorus. Cress tea is a natural blood purifier and is excellent for clearing the complexion and brightening the eyes. Apart from making one more robust, cress tea is said to help prevent hair from falling out. Parsley leaf tea combines well with cress leaf tea.

Dill seed tea
Dill seed tea is made in the same way as other seed teas. It is especially good for soothing wind and colic in babies, and in days gone by chemists used to stock a stabilised version, which was called "dill water". Given in *very weak* proportions in boiled water, this is a time-honoured remedy for young children. Dill tea helps the digestion and dispels flatulence. It is also reputed to strengthen the fingernails.

Elderflower Tea
The most popular elder tree grown in gardens is usually *Sambucus aurea* which has decorative golden leaves and the same type of flat, creamy blossoms as the true elder, *S. nigra,* or black elder, so called because of the plain, dark green of the foliage. Flowers from the latter are considered more efficacious for health than those of the golden elder. A tea made from the fresh or dried blooms is an old remedy for influenza. It was also taken every morning during the spring as a medicine for purifying the blood.

Elderflowers also have many cosmetic uses (see page 98), and they give a delicate flavour to certain foods, especially to a water ice (see page 124). If making tea or an infusion, follow the directions for flower teas on page 87.

Fennel seed tea
The most effective part of the fennel plant medicinally is the seeds, and the tea is made in exactly the same way as all the other seed teas. As well as relieving indigestion and helping to rid the body of uncomfortable gases, cooled fennel seed tea is excellent for bathing sore eyes. A strong infusion may be blended with honey and yoghurt and spread on the face and neck. Leave for fifteen minutes while you lie down with soaked cotton wool pads of the tea on your eyelids, then gently rinse off with tepid water. This treatment will leave the complexion smooth and clear and brighten the eyes.

Garlic
Is not recommended as a tea, its flavour is too pronounced, and there are other ways of using its remarkably effective qualities, as described on page 54.

Horseradish
Like garlic, is such a strongly flavoured herb that a tea of it would be unpalatable. Once again, there are other ways of making use of its properties and these are described on page 56.

Lemongrass leaf tea
This is one of the most palatable of all herb teas and is recommended as an introduction to herbal beverages. Being rich in vitamin A in a water soluble form it has the effect of clearing the skin and refining its texture.

Lime flower tea or linden tea

The fresh or dried flowers from the large lime tree, *Tilia europaea,* are used and it is traditional in Europe to take this tea for calming the nerves and to soothe the mucous linings following a head cold. This delicately fragrant tea is an excellent general tonic, and it may be taken regularly. Make the tea in the way described for flower teas at the beginning of this chapter.

Lovage leaf tea

Lovage tea, made from the fresh or dried leaves, stimulates the digestive organs. The strained, cooled tea is a soothing lotion for sore eyes. An infusion of the root is sometimes used for jaundice and bladder problems. A tea made from the seeds is recommended as a gargle for infections of the mouth and throat.

Marjoram and Oregano leaf tea

Marjoram and oregano tea is helpful at the onset of a fever because it induces perspiration. It also relieves colds, cramps, digestive troubles, nervous headaches and stomach pains. When mixed with chamomile flowers (which should be treated in the same way as the leaves) it acts as a tonic, as well as being soothing. A strong tea of the leaves, cooled and used as a final rinse, will help darken the hair of brunettes.

Mint leaf tea

Peppermint tea is possibly the best known of mint teas. Its medicinal value is in its purported ability to disperse congestion in the body, and to relieve indigestion, bronchitis, headaches, coughs and colds. It is delicious and healthful when taken icy cold in the summer, and is refreshing and revitalising on a hot day. Peppermint tea in double strength, cooled, and used as a hair rinse helps condition oily hair. Mint tea (made from spearmint leaves) is especially refreshing in very hot and humid weather. It is also good for the digestion and excellent for helping to dispel stomach gases; it cleanses the intestines, thus helping to overcome bad breath.

Nettle leaf tea

The dried leaves of the common nettle weed, *Urtica dioica,* are widely used by natural therapists. Julius Caesar is reputed to have introduced it to Britain. The tea contains vitamin D, iron, calcium and other important trace elements and is used as a spring tonic for the blood. It is taken in cases of arterial degeneration, rheumatism, gout and shortness of breath. The leaves, fresh or dried, make a delicious and nutritious soup.

Parsley leaf tea

Parsley is a very nutritious herb, containing vitamins A, B and C, as well as organic iron, potassium, silicon, magnesium and other trace elements. This tea assists the bladder, kidneys and liver, and is excellent for people suffering from anaemia. It is also helpful, together with other treatment, in overcoming chronic cystitis. It stimulates the appetite and is a tonic and cleansing tea. Parsley and watercress tea blend well with one another. One herbalist warns that pregnant women should avoid it. Cooled parsley tea may be rubbed into the hair before shampooing to make it shiny. Pads of cotton wool soaked in the cooled tea and patted on the skin close enlarged pores, freshen the skin and reduce puffiness around the eyes.

Raspberry leaf tea
This tea is made from dried raspberry leaves and has traditionally been given to expectant mothers. It has the reputation of easing childbirth and the expulsion of the afterbirth, as well as assisting lactation and hastening convalescence. It is soothing, tones up the mucous membranes, allays nausea, and encourages good bowel action.

Rose-hip tea
This beverage is very popular as a preventative against colds, being an excellent source of vitamin C, as well as vitamins A, E and B. The ripe fruits (hips) of wild roses are harvested, dried and shredded. To make the tea, use one teaspoonful for each cup, pour boiling water over it, allow to infuse, then strain. It can be taken hot in the winter with a slice of lemon, a little honey and a pinch of spice, or iced in summer with sprigs of mint, or peppermint, honey, ice cubes and lemon slices. Hibiscus flowers are often blended with rose-hip tea for "fragrant enjoyment".

Rosemary leaf tea
This tea is recommended for strengthening the memory and relieving headaches. It is a nerve tonic as well, and aids the digestion and kidneys. The cooled tea rubbed into the scalp is one of the best hair tonics, and used frequently will help the hair to become lustrous and dandruff-free. Make a stronger brew for this, as explained in the section on medicinal uses for rosemary.

Sage leaf tea
Sage tea is one of the most venerable: the ancient Egyptians and Chinese were aware of this. It is recognised as promoting longevity, strengthening the memory and restoring acuteness to the senses. It has a tonic effect on the liver, brain and nerves. It is an excellent tea when blended with balm. The cooled tea makes a soothing mouth rinse for inflamed gums, and is helpful as a gargle for sore throats. A stronger brew, cooled, may also be rubbed into the hair to prevent it from going grey. As well, cotton wool soaked in the cooled tea and patted gently on to the skin will help close enlarged pores.

Savory leaf tea
Both winter and summer savory make pleasant-tasting teas; either the fresh or dried leaves may be used. The tea is used to treat colic, flatulence, giddiness and respiratory troubles. Savory is an intestinal antiseptic and is also said to be an aphrodisiac!

Slippery elm bark tea
The highly nutritious bark comes from a small tree, *Ulmus fulva,* native to the United States and Canada. The only part used is the inner bark which is stripped and collected from the trunk and larger branches: it is dried and then powdered. When brewed into a beverage, or "gruel", it is very glutinous and can be difficult to become used to; however its powers of soothing the intestines, and its strengthening, healing and very nutritious qualities make it worth persevering with. To make it, put a teaspoon of the powder into a cup, mix it with a pinch of cinnamon and then add a little cold

water to make a paste. Pour on very hot water, or milk, stirring vigorously, and add a teaspoon of clear honey. The mixture will be rather thick and smoothly gelatinous (if it goes lumpy push it through a fine sieve) and this is the reason why it is so healing for the mucous membrane of the stomach and intestines. When taken before going to bed this draught will induce sleep. Although slippery elm is available in tablet form, we don't think it is quite as effective as the liquid.

Tarragon leaf tea
Herbalists recommend tarragon tea to ease indigestion and flatulence and, by acting as a diuretic, helps to rid the body of excess fluids.

Thyme leaf tea
Take this tea as an aid to digestion and to tone up the nervous system and respiratory organs; it is also an intestinal antiseptic, and has a delicious savoury flavour. The cooled tea used as a mouth rinse freshens the breath. Cotton wool dipped into the cooled tea and patted on to the skin helps to freshen and clear the complexion.

Valerian root tea
This tea has remarkable sedative properties and soothes and calms the nerves, without being habit-forming. It also relieves migraine and heart palpitations and is derived from the plant *Valerian officinalis*. It should be taken just before going to bed. Some herbal therapists advise that this tea should not be taken by people suffering from liver complaints as it can cause nausea.

Valerian tea has the reputation of having an unpleasant smell, so either mix it with a very pleasant tea, for instance lemongrass, or lace it well with honey and fresh fruit juice.

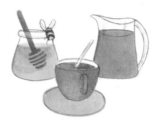

There are many other medicinal herb teas which would take a whole book of their own to write about. Those we have selected are brewed from the culinary, wholesome herbs written about in this book, with the addition of a few that are used for teas or "coffees", and which are readily obtainable from most specialist shops.

Dandelion coffee
This beverage is made from the roots of wild dandelions, *Taraxacum officinale,* as mentioned in the opening chapter of this section. It is sold by health food shops already packaged and ground to a powder, or in a granulated form. Some manufacturers use unnecessary additives, so try and make sure that the one you buy is made from pure dandelion root. Some brands, however, are blended with another *natural* product – which should be marked on the label – to make it more palatable because, on its own, dandelion coffee can be rather bitter for some tastes. This beverage acts as a tonic and stimulates the functions of the liver and urinary organs, which is why it helps to prevent rheumatism and similar complaints.

Delicious and Beneficial Orange Cordial

"6 or 8 oranges, 2 lemons, 2.5 kg (5 lb) sugar, 1.8 litres (3 pints) boiling water, 60 g (2 oz) tartaric acid, 30 g (1 oz) citric acid, 30 g (1 oz) Epsom salts. Pour boiling water over the juice and grated rinds and other ingredients. Stand until cold, then bottle. Keep a long time." From the C.W.A.'s *Coronation Cookery Book*.

N.B. I have made this concentrated cordial many times, and it is an excellent substitute for supermarket drinks, especially during school holidays when children have a never-ending thirst. Put 1 tablespoon of the cordial in a glass, fill with iced water (or mineral water for grown-ups) and ice. For guests, garnish with a sprig of spearmint or leafy sticks of eau-de-Cologne mint or peppermint. We usually store the concentrated orange cordial in bottles in the refrigerator to help its keeping qualities, and for extra chill when drinking it.

Mint Julep

"Wash a large bunch of mint, then place it in a basin and cover with 1 cup of sugar and the strained juice of 5 lemons. Leave for 2 hours, then transfer the liquid to a glass jug. Add a large lump of ice, 2 bottles of ginger ale and fresh sprigs of mint." From *The Coronation Cookery Book*.

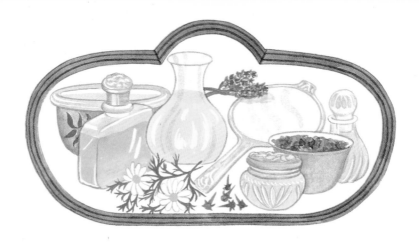

HERBS
FOR
BEAUTY

Since time immemorial men and women have adorned their bodies with coloured stones, polished bone, and the like, and have used plant dyes on their faces and bodies to enhance their appearance. Today we wear jewellery and use make-up and try to make ourselves look as attractive as possible. Making the most of ourselves enhances our self-esteem, and a clean, glowing skin, bright eyes, shining hair and a healthy, cared-for body all create a pleasant impression. An awareness of the advantages of a healthy life-style and basic skin and hair care ought to be nurtured in the young so that as they grow older these attributes, together with the self-assurance and wisdom gained through the experience of living, will give them added appeal.

There are many natural and inexpensive ways to beauty, and in the fol-lowing recipes we suggest just a few. Different herbs have various components which are helpful for skin, hair, teeth and eyes, and some of the foods we eat also have these properties so that they, too, can be used as beauty products. Some dairy products, fruits, vegetables and other natural foods, which also assist surface skin function, are excellent rejuvenating sources from the outside as well as from within. There are stories of how the legendary Cleopatra bathed in asses' milk to keep herself beautiful. Venetian ladies dyed their hair with saffron and henna (a natural substance) for golden or auburn locks. Kohl, mainly composed of powdered minerals, was introduced in Neolithic times and became an early Egyptian cosmetic for the eyes; nowadays it is used in a more refined form as an eyeliner. One of the latest beauty and health phenomena to re-emerge from ancient times is aloe vera *(Aloe barbadenisis)*, a native of North Africa and the Mediterranean region of southern Europe; it was known to the ancient Egyptians and is recorded in the Ebers Papyrus of 1500 B.C.

Facial Steaming

Herbal facial steaming is a well-tried and proven aid to a fresher, clearer skin. Dry skin brushing on the body is important too as a daily routine; for this, a long-handled brush, especially made for the purpose, is used. Brushing removes dead skin cells, eliminates acid, stimulates circulation and helps to maintain the body skin's elasticity. Inner cleansing is also important for a glowing skin and clear, sparkling eyes. Apart from drinking at least six glasses of water a day, and ensuring regular, complete, bowel evacuation by eating foods high in dietary fibre, certain herbs are particularly helpful for a clear skin. Lemongrass, for example, taken as a tea or in tablet form, is good, and garlic, eaten either raw or in the form of garlic oil capsules, which can be bought with the addition of parsley to make them odourless, is another.

For a herbal facial steam, the herbs or flowers are simmered in water so that the volatile essences and the medicating, cleansing properties are released. Steaming with herbs induces perspiration, which deep cleanses the pores of the skin, helps to eradicate blackheads, and improves circulation. As well, the facial tissues absorb moisture which has the effect of "plumping up" the skin. After steaming the face, the skin should be rinsed with warm water, gently patted with cotton wool soaked in a cold herb tea to close the pores, and then lightly dried. Allow an hour after a steam treatment for the pores to close completely before going outside. There are various steams to use for different types of skins, but the basic method of preparation is the same.

Thoroughly cleanse the skin before starting the treatment. Now put 2 tablespoons of fresh herb leaves or flowers (1 tablespoon if using the dried) into 5 cups (1.25 litres) of water in a saucepan (not aluminium) and, with the lid on, slowly bring to boiling point. Lower the heat and simmer the liquid for 2-3 minutes. Turn off the heat, put the saucepan onto a flat surface and remove the lid. Cover your hair with a shower cap, or wrap it in a towel, envelop your head and the saucepan with a towel and lower your face over the saucepan to within about 200 mm (8 inches). Close your eyes and let the steam circulate around your face by turning your head from side to side. If your skin is fine, or if you have close surface veins, 5 minutes should be enough. If you have broken veins, do not attempt a facial steam; instead, try cooled, soothing herb teas made from comfrey leaves, comfrey root, chamomile flowers or elder flowers applied to the face with cotton wool. For normal skins, allow 10 minutes' steaming. One or two facial steam treatments a week should be enough, as too many may destroy the skin's natural moisture and oils.

Here are some suggestions for facial steams according to skin type:

Normal to Dry Skins
Chopped comfrey leaves, chopped comfrey root and whole chamomile flowers mixed in equal quantities to make 2 tablespoons. Add to 5 cups (1.25 litres) of water and follow the general directions given above.

Normal to Oily Skins
Chopped comfrey leaves and comfrey root, chopped lemongrass, crushed fennel seeds and crumbled lavender flowers mixed in equal quantities to make 2 tablespoons. Add to 5 cups (1.25 litres) of water and follow the general directions given above.

Problem Skins
To help overcome acne, try chopped comfrey root, crumbled lavender flowers and chopped lemongrass mixed in equal quantities to make 2 tablespoons. Add to 5 cups (1.25 litres) of water and follow the general directions given above.

To Tighten and Stimulate the Skin
Chopped peppermint leaves, chopped comfrey leaves, crushed aniseed and rosemary leaves mixed in equal quantities to make 2 tablespoons. Add to 5 cups (1.25 litres) of water and follow the general directions given above.

To Moisturise and Soothe the Skin
Chopped orange peel, whole orange blossoms, chopped comfrey root and crushed fennel seeds mixed in equal quantities to make 2 tablespoons. Add to 5 cups (1.25 litres) of water and follow the general directions given above.

Beauty Treatments

Fresh Strawberry Mask
An old beauty treatment for refreshing and revitalising the skin was to apply a mask of fresh strawberries to the face and neck. After cleansing the skin, or after a facial steam, cut up and mash to a pulp enough strawberries to spread all over the face and neck, leaving the eye area clear. Lie down for 20 minutes. For extra benefit, soak cotton-wool pads in a cold tea made from crushed fennel seeds and put them on your closed eyelids. Rinse the mask off with warm water, then splash cold water all over the face and neck.

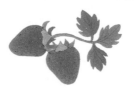

Elderflower Lotion for Sunburn and Freckles
This is very easy to make and does wonders for any skin, especially if used regularly for several weeks. Not only does it soothe sunburn and eliminate some of the redness, it also fades freckles and gives the complexion a fine-textured lustre. Men can use this as a soothing aftershave lotion, and it also alleviates tired or sore eyes.

We have made this lotion with dried elderflowers, and if you have a tree (*Sambucus nigra*) you can collect the heads of frothy, creamy blossoms and use them fresh; or dry them on sheets of paper in a dry, airy place until they shrivel into fragile, filigree-flowers, the colour of old ivory, then store them in airtight containers.

Pour 2 cups (16 fl oz) boiling water onto 2 tablespoons of crumbled, fresh elderflowers or 1 tablespoon fragmented, dried elderflowers. Cover and leave for at least 15 minutes, then strain the lotion into a screw-top jar and store in the refrigerator. (Otherwise it will develop an unpleasant odour.) Instead of washing your face in the morning, pour some elderflower lotion into a small bowl, and, with cotton wool, pat it all over the face and neck and allow it to dry on the skin. This quantity should be enough for one week if the lotion is kept in a cold place, and it will stay fresh enough to use for that length of time.

Elderflower for the Eyes
Make an infusion as described above, but be sure to strain it through fine muslin or cheesecloth before using. Bathe the eyes several times a day with the lotion.

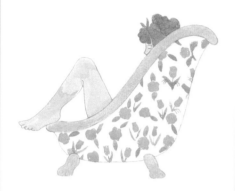

Scented Baths

A Cosmetic Bath
Take two pounds of Barley or Bean-meal, eight pounds of Bran, and a few handfuls of Borage leaves. Boil these ingredients in a sufficient quantity of spring water. Nothing cleanses and softens the skin like this Bath.
"The Toilet of Flora", from *The Scented Garden* by E. S. Rohde.

An Aromatic Bath
Boil, for the space of two or three minutes, in a sufficient quantity of river water, one or more of the following plants; viz. Laurel, Thyme, Rosemary, Wild Thyme, Sweet Marjoram, Bastard-Marjoram, Lavender, Southernwood, Wormwood, Sage, Pennyroyal, Sweet-Basil, Balm, Wild Mint, Hyssop, Clove-july-flowers, Anise, Fennel, or any other herbs that have an agreeable scent. Having strained off the liquor from the herbs, add to it a little Brandy, or camphorated Spirits of Wine.
From *The Scented Garden* by E. S. Rohde.

Jasmine Oil
Nothing more is required than to dip the finest cotton wool in clear olive oil, which must be spread in thin layers, in a tall glass vessel, with alternate layers of Jessamine flowers which, in a few days, will impart the whole of their perfume to the cotton. The oil may then be pressed out for use: and the cotton itself may be laid in drawers or band-boxes, where its perfume is wished for.
"Practical Economy (1822)" From *The Scented Garden* by E. S. Rohde.

Flower-scented Facial Cleansing Oil

1 cup olive oil
1 tablespoon avocado oil
1/2 cup (4 fl oz) apricot kernel oil
1/2 cup (4 fl oz) walnut oil
1/4 teaspoon essential flower oil (e.g. lavender, rose, jasmine, violet, lotus, or ylang ylang – available from specialist herbal shops)

Pour all the oils into a screw-top jar and shake it vigorously. Store in the refrigerator. To use, pour some of the oil onto a piece of cotton wool and gently apply to the face and neck until clean, using an outward and upward movement. Remove oily residue with an alcohol-free toning lotion, or witch-hazel, by pouring a little onto slightly damp cotton wool, and using the same upward and outward motion. Use this cleanser to remove make-up, city smog, perspiration, and so on.

Honey and Milk Rejuvenating Lotion

1 cup (8 fl oz) clear honey
1/2 cup (4 fl oz) milk
2 teaspoons rosewater (available from a
chemist or continental delicatessen)

Warm the honey gently in a saucepan. Add the milk and rosewater, turning off the heat at the same time. Stir until the ingredients are amalgamated. Allow to cool, then pour the lotion into a container and store it in the refrigerator. Before using, stir again if the mixture has separated, and pour a little into a saucer. Soak cotton wool balls in the lotion and pat onto the face and neck. Use this lotion every night and do not rinse it off until the next morning.

Avocado Face and Neck Freshener

Avocado oil is an excellent moisturiser to use under make-up, particularly in drying winds. Fresh avocado on the face and neck is especially nourishing for the skin.

Scoop out the flesh from half an avocado and mash it to a pulp. Spread the pulp on the face and neck and lie down, if possible, for 20 minutes. Remove with tissues, then dampened cotton wool.

Herbal Aftershave Lotion

1 tablespoon chopped sage leaves
1 tablespoon chopped comfrey leaves
1 tablespoon rosemary leaves
1 1/2 cups (12 fl oz) apple cider vinegar
1 1/2 cups (12 fl oz) witch-hazel

Put the herbs and vinegar into a stoppered glass jar and stand it on a sunny windowsill to infuse for 1 week. Strain, then stir in the witch-hazel. Store in an airtight container in the refrigerator.

Rosemary Hair Rinse

Shampoos and hair lotions containing pure extract of rosemary will revitalise the scalp and hair and will help to prevent dandruff. Herbal cosmetic manufacturers produce these shampoos and conditioners, but if you have a rosemary bush in the garden you will be able to make this simple lotion yourself.

Gather about 4-6 leafy rosemary stalks and simmer them in 5 cups (1.25 litres) of water for 30 minutes. Keep the lid on the saucepan to prevent the precious vapour from evaporating. Strain and cool, then use as a final rinse after washing your hair, rubbing the lotion well into the scalp.

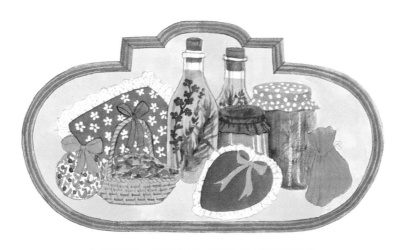

HERBS
AS
GIFTS

Many charming, unique and useful gifts may be made from herbs and flowers. Always appreciated are piquant, aromatic herb vinegars, delectable jams and jellies fragrant with roses or scented herb leaves, preserved sugary flowers and savoury, crumbled "bouquet garnis" rolled into small cheesecloth or calico balls tied with string for casseroles, soups or stews.

Hair rinses, lotions for the face and other cosmetics are made with bounty gathered from the garden. Nostalgic perfumes of leaves and blossoms, redolent of glowing sunlit gardens, are evoked by various types of potpourris. Exotic scents of the East are contained in a spicy pomander ball. Among many other delights are herbal "bath balls" for tying under a hot running tap, "moth bags" containing a special mixture of sweet and bitter herbs and pungent spices to repel unwanted marauders in cupboards and drawers, and of course, lavender sachets, forever a beloved favourite. Sleep pillows filled with soothing lavender, balmy lemon verbena, and gentle rose petals release a mingling of Nature's tender opiates for untroubled slumber.

In the garden at night

"Be still, my soul. Consider
The flowers and the stars.
Among these sleeping fragrances,
Sleep now your cares.
That which the universe
Lacks room to enclose
Lives in the folded petals
Of this dark rose."

Gerald Bullet (From *A Gift of Flowers* by Frances Berrill and Helen Exley. Angus and Robertson.)

Crystallised flowers

Attractively packaged and ribbon-tied crystallised flowers or fragrant leaves make an unusual and most acceptable gift. The sugared confections can be put on top of whipped cream as a finishing touch to a special dessert, or on trifles, on cake icings, and any other special gastronomical treat.

The following is the simplest and quickest way to crystallise flowers. Whole small blooms or single petals may be used, the most suitable being violets, borage flowers, rosemary flowers, English primroses, rose petals, small, whole rosebuds, and jasmine flowers. The various scented mint leaves are excellent too.

Put the white of an egg into a saucer, break it up with a fork, but do not whip it. Take a dry flower, or a single petal, and with a small paint brush dipped into the egg white, cover it completely. Then shake caster sugar through a fine sieve over the flower, first on one side, then the other. As each is finished, place on greaseproof paper laid in a small ovenproof dish. Put the flowers in a very slow oven with the door open for approximately 10-15 minutes, gently turning them as the sugar glazes and hardens. Do not leave too long or they will go brown. Store the candied flowers (or leaves) between layers of greaseproof paper in an airtight box. (From *The Lansdowne Book of Herbs and Spices,* by John and Rosemary Hemphill.)

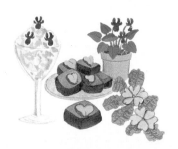

Rose-Petal Jam

A small glass jar, or a special pottery bowl, filled with fragrant rose-petal jam, is a very special and quite exotic gift. Use the jam to spoon over ice-cream, or to spread on thin, crustless triangles of bread and butter, or on hot, buttered scones.

To 50 fully opened, fragrant red (or red and pink together) roses, allow 4 litres (2 pints) of water and 1.5 kg (3 lb) of caster (powdered) sugar. Boil the sugar and water until it is slightly candied. Add the juice of a lemon and the rose petals, which have been gently pulled from the flowers. Stir well and bring to the boil. Put in a pat of unsalted butter to clear the scum and then simmer for approximately one hour. It is necessary to stir frequently, every five minutes or so, or the colour will be brown instead of a translucent, ruby red. Cool, pour into clean pots or jars, and cover when cold.

If the mixture seems a little too thin, add some fruit pectin (available from health food shops or grocers), following the instructions on the packet.

Clove Apple (or Orange)

To keep away moths

It is important to start with a fresh, firm apple, or a ripe, fresh, thin skinned orange. Stick the fruit full of cloves, starting from the stalk end and going around as many times as is needed to cover it, leaving a small space between each clove. Now roll the fruit well in 2 teaspoons of orris root powder and 2 teaspoons of ground cinnamon mixed together. Wrap the fruit in tissue paper and put it away in a dark cupboard for a few weeks. A staple may be pressed into the top at this stage so that when the fruit has hardened, ribbon may be threaded through it. Alternatively, ribbon can be passed around the fruit four times, giving a "basket" effect, and then more ribbon can be attached to the top so that the clove apple can be hung from a coat-hanger in a wardrobe, or, using a pretty idea from the past, on a door-handle. Velvet or corded ribbon in colourful shades makes a charming contrast with the snuff-brown of the pomander. Once the fruit has hardened, it will last indefinitely, gradually shrinking over a period of time. We do not know what happens to the inside. We once broke one open, using a cleaver because it was iron-hard, and there was no sign of anything at all, not even a pip!

Peppermint-Geranium Jelly

This is another unusual and delicious-tasting conserve that will make a unique and very special gift. Other types of scented geranium leaves may be used instead.

1 small bunch stalkless peppermint-geranium leaves (about 1 cup)
5 cups (2 lbs) caster (powdered) sugar
juice of 2 small lemons or 1 large lemon
4 cups (1 litre) water
125 g (4 oz) powdered pectin
green food colouring or
Crème de Menthe

Wash the geranium leaves and steep them in the sugar and lemon juice for one hour. Place in a saucepan with the water and bring to the boil. Strain, add the pectin (follow the instructions on the package), and boil again, stirring for about a minute. Add the food colouring or Crème de Menthe. Pour into clean jars or pots, placing a small peppermint-geranium leaf in each one. Seal the lids. This will keep in the refrigerator for several weeks.

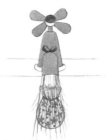

Bath Sachets
Soothing Lavender

These are made with the dried flowers of English lavender. French lavender flowers may be used instead but they do not have the highly incensed perfume of English lavender. The sticky, oily leaves of French lavender give an excellent, strong fragrance. Both of these lavenders soothe the nerve-endings of the body, and the best way to do this is to lie in a bath permeated with the essential oils, either released from the bath sachets or from drops of the essential oil, or a lavender "bath milk". (Smelling lavender flowers for some time when packaging it acts as a soporific.)

As these sachets are disposable after several uses, do not buy expensive material for them; select a pretty, sprigged, thin cotton, or other suitable fabric in lavender colours.

Cut the fabric into small squares, put a small pile of lavender in the middle and tie into a ball, securing it with a long piece of string; use pinking shears to prevent fraying. Tie about six together with a lavender-coloured bow and attach a little card, saying: "Soothing Lavender Bath Sachets: tie to the hot tap and run hot water over the sachet to release the natural essences. May be used two or three times."

Revitalising rosemary
Use the same idea for rosemary bath sachets, which, instead of being sleep-

inducing, are revitalising. A rosemary bath is an excellent way to start the day, or before going out again at night. For these sachets use green or blue sprigged material since rosemary flowers are blue.

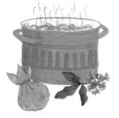

Bouquet Garni

This is a useful gift for people who like to use a *bouquet garni* in little sachets, which are removed after cooking. Buy, or make, a *bouquet garni* of crumbled, dried bay leaves, dried thyme, dried marjoram and dried parsley. Put a little pile of the herbs in the middle of a muslin square and tie with a long piece of string for easy removal at the end of the cooking time. Put about six sachets into a celluloid box, or a cellophane bag, attractively tied with ribbon.

Herb Vinegars

There are many different uses for the herbs in your garden, so while they are still bountiful, making herb vinegars is a very satisfying and useful task, and they make delightful and unusual gifts. The vinegar may be flavoured with various herbs, or a combination of compatible-tasting herbs. Tarragon, rosemary, savory, basil, thyme, marjoram, oregano, garlic and lemon balm, as well as dill and mint, all make strongly flavoured vinegars on their own. Parsley and fennel combine well, as do parsley and peppercorns, or parsley and garlic. Rose-petal vinegar is an unusual and colourful vinegar with several uses.

Herb vinegars make delicious vinaigrette dressings. One tablespoon of herb vinegar to three tablespoons of oil is the usual mixture. There are many interesting oils on the market, as well as the time-honoured olive oil. A few to choose from are walnut oil hazelnut oil, apricot-kernel oil, sunflower-seed oil, or pumpkin-seed oil. Some of these rather rare oils may only be available from specialist delicatessens or health food shops, but they are well worth ferreting out.

Making the vinegars is simple. Pick and wash the herbs to be used and dry them on absorbent paper. Pack the leaves into clean bottles or jars with lids, and fill with white wine vinegar, replacing the lids firmly. Another method is to heat the vinegar first to hasten the release of the oils from the leaves before pouring it over them. Stand the infusing vinegars on a sunny windowsill for about two weeks. The warmth from the sun releases the flavour and perfume of the herbs. If there is no sun during this time, let them stand for two more weeks. Some herbs lose their colour and become pallid-looking after soaking in the vinegar and giving out their colour and flavour. If this happens, strain the vinegar into a clean bottle and put in a fresh, washed sprig of the herb. This not only improves the appearance but adds flavour. Replace the lids and label the bottles. If using red rose petals, the vinegar will gradually turn a most beautiful rich crimson. This is a valuable ingredient for subtle salad dressings but may also be used to relieve headaches. An old remedy is to soak a cloth in the vinegar, wring it out and apply the wet cloth to the forehead. Repeat until the vinegar in the bowl is used up.

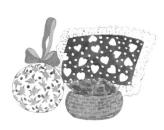

Potpourri

Making one's own potpourri is a delightfully nostalgic and soul satisfying occupation, as well as being very personal. Picking scented, colourful blooms and aromatic leaves from the garden, then drying them to capture the fragrances of spring, summer and autumn, then mixing them with other ingredients to complete the haunting bouquet, is a lasting reminder of glowing colours and delicately pervasive perfumes.

There are a host of different potpourris one can concoct, using various blossoms and foliage: the dried flowers from a wedding bouquet, or a posy from someone dear to you, can be preserved forever. Once the petals and leaves have been picked from their stems and thoroughly dried, all they need is the addition of appropriate essential oils, blended into orris powder, and a little spice to enhance the sweet flower scents. Orris powder is made from the ground, fragrant rhizome of the Florentine iris and its purpose is to "take up" the natural oils, and to keep the potpourri dry because it has a tendency to become mildewed in humid weather. Choosing the oils to complement the potpourri is a delightful task, especially as more is becoming known about aromatherapy (see page 81)

Sleep pillows, or dream pillows, are another kind of potpourri, and the herbs used in them fulfil various functions. Lavender is conducive to drowsiness, the Greeks believe that Lemon verbena brings sweet dreams, and rose petals are for harmony. Pillows filled with hops are also sleep inducing, although not sweet-smelling! We have come across 'aphrodisiac' sachets (perhaps these contain vervain, neroli, ylang ylang and marjoram), anti-sinus sachets, containing eucalyptus and pine but no orris powder – some people are allergic to orris.

Here is a list of some oils and their supposed influence on moods – an idea worth trying in various potpourris. For use as an inhalant or as a massage oil, or for burning as incense, choose only one oil at a time.

Concentration and willpower: bay, cedarwood, ginger, sage.
Meditation and tranquillity: bergamot, lavender, rose, sandalwood, patchouli, ylang ylang, jasmine.
Relaxation: coriander, lavender, pine, lemongrass.
Devotional: neroli, rose, ylang ylang, boronia, jasmine.
Psychic mood: bergamot, lavender, lemongrass, petitgrain, sandalwood, verbena.
Healing: bay, rose, sandalwood, wintergreen, mandarin.
Memory and mental stimulation: rosemary, pine, thyme, sage.
Weddings and festivities: neroli, rose, boronia, jasmine.
Femininity: bergamot, rose-geranium, lavender, rose, jasmine.
Masculinity: cedarwood, pine, ginger.
For soothing sleep: lavender, valerian, rose, lemon-verbena.
For clearing sinuses: pine, eucalyptus, rosemary.
(Some of the information about essential oils and their influence on moods is in Sally E. Janssen's excellent little book *Incense.*)

A lasting and fragrant potpourri

Potpourris made with ingredients that are easily available are just as successful and satisfying to make as those that contain "bay salt" (sea salt), which can make a potpourri mouldy in damp weather, or "gum benzoin", storax, civet, ambergris, and benjamin, all of which are unnecessary and not easily available.

If you have perfumed roses (especially red and pink ones) and lavender growing in the garden, as well as other fragrant flowers, including those of citrus-bearing trees like orange, cumquat and lemon, you have the beginnings of a potpourri. Other useful potpourri flowers that are easily grown in most home gardens are mignonette and jasmine, to name but a few, as well as perfumed foliage like lemon verbena, scented-leaved geraniums (especially rose-scented), and sweet-smelling herb leaves, such as eau-de-Cologne mint, which is delightful in a potpourri.

Aromatic spices are blended with the flowery and leafy scents to give a warmly contrasting and interesting depth to the blend, while powdered orris root 'takes up' the essential oils and distributes them through the mixture, at the same time preventing it from becoming moist and mildewed.

Essential oils help to preserve the fragrance of a potpourri. The choice of oils is personal, and they should be of top quality. One oil or three different ones can be blended into the orris powder but it is important that the oils should be complementary and not all of the same type; for instance, two sweet oils like rose and jasmine used together would be overpowering. Aim for a 'sharp' scent, use one oil that has a lingering perfume and another which is sweet. In time your sense of smell will be sharpened and become more selective. The oils suggested in the recipe are a guide only:

Sweet: lavender, jasmine, rose, lily-of-the-valley, violet.
Sharp: lemongrass, pine, rosemary, petitgrain, lemon (lavender has a sharpness underlying its sweetness).
Lingering: cedarwood, clove, rose-geranium, musk, sandalwood.

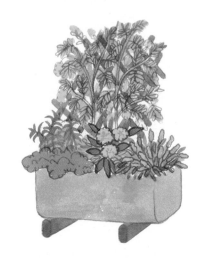

Method

Gather the flowers and leaves in dry weather early in the day, before the sun has become too hot, then spread them out to dry on racks or sheets of newspaper in a shady, airy place. (Scented leaves should be cut away from the stems for quicker drying.) A microwave oven can be used for drying potpourri ingredients and this method is described on page 23. When crisp-dry, measure the flowers and leaves (large leaves like peppermint-geranium should be crunched by hand into fairly small pieces), and put them into an earthenware or glass container with a lid.

For 4 cups of dried material you will need 1 tablespoon of orris powder, 1 teaspoon of each of the chosen oils, and 1 teaspoon of ground cinnamon.

Mix the orris powder and cinnamon, then add the oils and mix well. Sprinkle this crumbly mixture over the dried flowers and leaves, stir well, put the lid on the container and leave for 2-3 weeks, stirring occasionally. The blend is now ready to be put into one large decorative bowl, or into several smaller ones. Alternatively, you can use small pottery or stoneware jars or pomanders, or you could make attractive sachets from pieces of fabric such as muslin, voile, cambric, organdie, and the like. Small plastic boxes with colourful leaves and flowers look charming and cost very little. (The box is pierced to release the fragrance.) Even cellophane paper bags can be used. Pieces of cinnamon bark, whole cloves, bay leaves and dried strips of orange or lemon peel are all excellent additions to a potpourri mixture.

N.B. Do not expect to have all the flowers and leaves ready at the same time. It is usual to collect and dry them while they are at their peak, and when you have the time, and then to store them in covered containers until you are ready to make the potpourri. You can always add to the potpourri, even after several weeks, provided the ingredients are dry, except for the oils, of course, which will have to be mixed with a little more orris powder before adding to the fragrant pot.

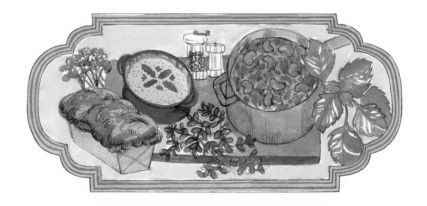

COOKING
WITH
HERBS

The following recipes contain ingredients which are not unusual in everyday cooking except for the inclusion of certain herbs or edible flowers. These give flavour, colour, nourishment, digestive qualities for easier assimilation, and piquancy to the palate.

It is astounding how the varied tastes of herbs can alter the character of any dish, and experimenting is always recommended. However, there are excellent traditional reasons for combining many foods and herbs. For instance, some herb seeds (which are usually listed as spices once they are dried) have remarkably therapeutic digestive-aiding oils locked into them, like dill seeds, caraway seeds, fennel seeds, coriander seeds, anise seeds (aniseed) and cardamom seeds. Some are incorporated into special recipes for helping to dispel flatulence . . . cab-

bage dishes with dill or caraway seeds, starchy yeast cookery with any of the above seeds and succulent, fatty pork, duck, or goose with dry, aromatic sage leaves to counteract too much richness, are some examples.

The use of a special herb, or a combination of herbs, occurs in various recipes, and in the chapter *All About Herbs* we have given their medicinal and culinary properties, so that the reasons for using them in a given dish are clear. Once again, a favourite herb flavour of your own choice should, through testing, be tried as well.

The employment of fragrant, silky-petalled flowers is a nutritious, delicate way of sampling some of the rarefied essences within the heart of blooms, usually only enjoyed by butterflies and bees.

"Cookery . . . means the knowledge of all herbs and fruits and balms and spices, and all that is healing and sweet in the fields and groves, and savoury in meats..." (Part of a quotation by Ruskin from *The Gentle Art of Cookery* by Mrs. C. F. Leyel and Miss Olga Hartley, Chatto and Windus, London, 1925. The original book was given to us many years ago by a very old lady to whom it belonged, and is now available again in paperback with a foreword by Elizabeth David.)

Parsley Soup

Serves 6

This is an excellent and nourishing soup, rich in vitamins.

1 large bunch of parsley
 (about 125 g/4 oz)
500 g (1 lb) potatoes
½ lettuce
1 medium-sized white onion
2 teaspoons salt
8 cups (2 litres) water

Wash the parsley, reserve a little for garnishing, and cut the rest up coarsely, removing the stalks. Peel and wash the potatoes; cut into small chunks. Wash the lettuce, discarding any discoloured leaves, and chop roughly. Peel onion. Put all these ingredients into a large saucepan with the salt and water, and bring to the boil. Simmer with the lid on for 45 minutes to 1 hour. Purée the slightly cooled soup in a blender, or press soup through a sieve. Return to the saucepan to reheat. Garnish each serving with the reserved parsley, either chopped or in small, whole sprigs, and serve hot. In summer, chill the soup and add a spoonful of sour cream to each serving before decorating with the parsley.

Mrs Goddard's Chervil and Avocado Soup

Serves 6
2 medium-sized ripe avocados
1 clove garlic, crushed
1 tablespoon lemon juice
2½ cups (20 fl oz) cold chicken stock
salt
freshly ground black pepper
1¼ cups (10 fl oz) sour cream
1 tablespoon chopped chervil
 (or 2 teaspoons chopped green dill)

Halve the avocados, remove the stones and set them aside, scoop out the flesh, including all the green part next to the skin. Chop the flesh roughly and purée in a blender at high speed with the garlic, lemon juice, half the stock, salt and pepper. Pour the mixture into a large bowl and stir in the cream and the remainder of the stock; whisk until blended. Fold in the chervil, add the stones (to prevent discoloration), cover and chill for 2 hours. Garnish with a small spray of chervil (or dill) and serve with a slice of lemon and an ice cube in each bowl. Accompany the soup with Prawn and Parsley Rolls (page 112).

Pumpkin and Basil Soup

Serves: 6
1 kg (2 lb) pumpkin, peeled and roughly chopped
2 potatoes, peeled and roughly chopped
1 onion, chopped
1 tablespoon chopped basil
salt and pepper
2 chicken stock cubes
5 cups (1.25 litres) water
sour cream

Boil all ingredients (except sour cream) until tender. Cool and purée. Return the soup to the saucepan and simmer for 30 minutes until thick. Serve with sour cream.

Lovage Soup

Serves: 4

30 g (1 oz) butter or vegetable margarine
2 tablespoons wholemeal flour
2½ cups (20 fl oz) chicken stock (may be made with stock cubes)
½ cup (4 fl oz) milk
1 tablespoon chopped lovage leaves
2 teaspoons lemon juice
salt
1 tablespoon chopped chives
yoghurt or sour cream

Melt the butter in a saucepan, add the flour and blend to a smooth paste. Gradually pour in the warmed stock, stirring until thickened. Still stirring, add the milk, lovage and lemon juice. Simmer for 15 to 20 minutes and add the salt. Purée the soup and return it to the saucepan. Stir in the chives and cook for a few minutes only.

Serve either hot or chilled and garnish with a swirl of plain yoghurt or sour cream, topped with a sprig of fresh lovage.

Crab Cocktail in Herb Yoghurt Sauce

Serves: 4

1 cup (8 oz) unflavoured yoghurt
1 tablespoon tomato paste
2 teaspoons finely chopped savory tops
2 teaspoons of either tarragon, dill, or chervil, finely chopped
2 teaspoons lemon juice
250 g (8 oz) crab, flaked (remove any sharp pieces)

Mix all the ingredients together, except the crab. Chill. Fold the crab into the sauce and serve in individual glasses garnished with a sprig of savory. An excellent accompaniment is thin brown bread crustless sandwiches filled with herbs.

Avocado, Cress and Caviare Mould

Serves 8

2 tablespoons gelatine melted in a little hot water – stir briskly until clear
3 avocados, peeled, stoned and sliced
1 tablespoon lemon juice
4 cups (1 litre) canned beef consommé
1 tablespoon finely chopped onion
3 tablespoons black lumpfish roe (often called caviare)
1 tablespoon chopped cress

Purée the avocados, lemon juice, consommé and onion in a blender or food processor until smooth. (Do it in batches so as not to overload the appliance.) Transfer the mixture to a bowl and fold in the gelatine mixture, lumpfish roe and cress. Pour into individual moulds, or a shallow dish, and leave to set in the refrigerator. To serve, unmould, or cut into squares, and accompany with sour cream and sprigs of cress.

Herb sandwiches

Fresh herb sandwiches are both nourishing and delicious. A thin coating of cream cheese or Vegemite (Marmite) on the bottom slice of buttered bread will help to bring out the flavour of the herbs without being overpowering. Unsalted, "sweet" butter is recommended, unless margarine is preferred. There are other spreads, or fillings, which seem to complement certain herbs, and some suggestions are given below. It is always interesting to experiment with flavour combinations too.

Herb sandwiches can be served for morning or afternoon tea – with cakes or biscuits as well if you wish – although most people nowadays prefer not to eat very much between meals, if at all, so herb sandwiches on their own are usually quite sufficient. They also make an excellent accompaniment to a first course.

Use a good quality fresh bread, either white or brown, and cut the slices as thin as possible. Butter the bread first, then cut through with a very sharp knife. Alternatively, sliced sandwich bread may be used. Cover the bottom slices with your chosen spread, then the chopped herbs, then close the sandwich. When enough have been made, remove the crusts and cut the sandwiches into triangles, squares, or fingers. (The smaller the better for a dinner party.) Put the sandwiches onto an attractive plate and cover with plastic film or foil and store in the refrigerator until needed. Alternatively, roll up each crustless slice of buttered, herb-strewn bread (the bread must be very fresh for this) and secure with a toothpick, which can be removed before serving.

The most delectable herb rolls we have tasted accompanied a first course of iced chervil and avocado soup, for lunch, in an English dining-room. We were seated at a gleaming table that reflected the gentle noon light filtering through scented wistaria hanging over open French doors leading to a rose garden. Kind friends had driven us from London to their country house on a warm spring day. Driving through the countryside, we passed lush green and golden fields shimmering in the sun and hedgerows thickly embroidered with starry-white Queen Anne's Lace, until we came to a story-book village, and the comfortable, old, elegant house where we were spoilt for the whole weekend. Soft feather beds enveloped us like cocoons at night. In the morning, the butler arrived with steaming cups of Earl Grey tea to awaken us, and Mrs Goddard, the housekeeper, plied us with the most delicious food. She very kindly gave us her recipe for Prawn and Parsley Rolls, and her Chervil and Avocado Soup is on page 109.

Fillings for herb sandwiches

- Thin slices of white, buttered bread, spread fairly thickly with cream cheese spread, and sprinkled with chopped garlic chives. (The late Claire Simpson's recipe.)
- Scrambled egg, cooled, mixed with a rasher of cooked, crumbled bacon and chopped fresh oregano.
- Swiss cheese slices scattered with chopped fresh, stalkless savory.
- A thin layer of Vegemite or Marmite, and stalkless, soft marjoram leaves, left whole.
- Crunchy peanut butter and chopped onion chives.
- Mashed banana mixed with lemon juice, sugar, cinnamon and chopped mint leaves between crisp lettuce leaves; eat soon after making.
- Thinly sliced, skinned (if preferred) tomato and chopped basil between crisp lettuce leaves. (The lettuce leaves form a barrier between the moist fillings and the bread, thus preventing the bread from becoming soggy.)
- Sliced cucumber, chopped dill or chervil, between crisp lettuce leaves.
- Salad sandwich – comprising a crisp lettuce leaf on the top and bottom slices of bread, alfalfa (or other) sprouts, thinly sliced tomato, grated carrot, finely chopped chives, and chopped (or whole) mint leaves.
- Cold chicken, sliced or chopped, and *fines herbes* (equal quantities of finely chopped parsley, chervil, chives and tarragon).
- Chopped cress, with or without cream cheese.
- Flaked salmon mixed with lemon juice and chopped tarragon or chervil.
- Chopped prawns with a squeeze of lemon juice and a sprinkling of *fines herbes*.
- Thinly sliced tongue and a scattering of very finely chopped
- Mashed liverwurst mixed with crumbled, cooked bacon and chopped sage leaves.

Mrs Goddard's Prawn and Parsley Rolls

Prepare thin, fresh, crustless brown bread slices, butter well, then cover with chopped prawns, roll firmly, wrap with plastic film and leave to 'set' in the refrigerator. (Use a toothpick to keep the shape if necessary.) To serve, dip each end of the rolls into melted butter, and then into finely chopped parsley, which will stick to the melted butter. This last step can be done in advance, the rolls covered with plastic film again and refrigerated before serving.

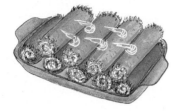

Gwennyth's Bran Muffins

2 cups (8 oz) unprocessed bran
1 cup (4 oz) wholemeal flour
1 teaspoon bicarbonate of soda
   (baking soda)
½ teaspoon baking powder
¾ cup golden (light corn) syrup,
   melted in 1 cup (8 fl oz) milk
1 teaspoon very finely chopped fresh
   rosemary leaves

In a bowl, combine bran and the flour sifted with the soda and baking powder. Fold in the melted golden syrup and milk mixture, then the rosemary, until well blended together. Spoon into buttered muffin pans and bake in a moderate oven for 15-20 minutes. Slice in half and serve buttered and hot, or warm.

Garlic Herb Bread

1 oblong loaf of rye bread
2 garlic cloves, crushed
1 tablespoon chopped parsley
1 tablespoon chopped marjoram
2 teaspoons chopped sage
1 teaspoon finely chopped thyme leaves
250 g (8 oz) butter or vegetable margarine,
softened

Using a sharp knife slice the bread thinly, almost to the bottom crust. Mash the garlic and herbs into the butter and spread generously on both sides of each bread slice. Wrap the loaf loosely in foil and put it in an ovenproof dish in a hot oven (230°C/450°F/Gas 8) for 10 to 15 minutes, until the bread is crisp. Serve hot.

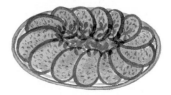

Tarragon Fish Pie

Serves 4-5
375 g (12 oz) cooked fish, flaked
1½ cups (12 oz) béchamel sauce
salt and pepper
1 scant tablespoon chopped tarragon
1 tablespoon walnut pieces, mixed with
   1 cup (2 oz) fresh brown breadcrumbs
butter, cubed

Stir the fish into the béchamel sauce. Season with salt and pepper to taste and add the tarragon. Pour into a buttered ovenproof dish, top with walnut and breadcrumb mixture and dot with the butter cubes. Heat through in a moderate oven until the breadcrumbs have browned. Serve with slices of lemon and very thin brown bread and butter, or herb sandwiches.

Elizabeth's Spinach Pie With Rosemary

Serves: 6 as an accompaniment
*   4 as a main dish*
1 bunch spinach (about 20 leaves)
2 teaspoons finely chopped rosemary leaves
1/2 cup (2 oz) fetta cheese, crumbled
1/2 teaspoon ground nutmeg
2 eggs, beaten
salt (optional, as fetta is very salty)
pepper
12 sheets filo pastry
1 tablespoon melted butter

Strip all green leaves from the spinach stalks (use the stalks in soup or a Chinese dish). Chop the leaves finely and put them into a saucepan with a little butter and the rosemary; steam lightly until cooked. Drain well in a colander, reserving some of the water. (When cooled, the spinach may be puréed in a blender with some of the reserved water for extra smoothness.)

Put the spinach and rosemary mixture into a bowl with the cheese, nutmeg and eggs; stir until well mixed. Transfer to a buttered ovenproof dish and cover with filo pastry using 2 sheets at a time and brushing with melted butter until all the pastry is used.

Bake in a moderately hot oven (180°C/350°F/Gas 4) until heated through and the pastry is brown and crisp. Eat while hot. Serve as an accompaniment to a main dish or as a light meal with hot buttered bread or rolls.

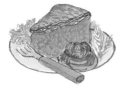

Cold Salmon Soufflé with Rosemary

Serves 4-6
1 1/2 cups (12 fl oz) beef consommé
1 tablespoon gelatine dissolved in a little
*   hot water*
150 ml (4 fl oz) thick mayonnaise
1 1/4 cups (10 fl oz) cream, whipped
2 teaspoons very finely chopped rosemary
500 g (1 lb), or nearest weight,
*   red salmon, flaked and bones removed*
1 small jar red lumpfish roe
*   (red "caviare")*

Put the consommé, dissolved gelatine and mayonnaise into a bowl and stir until well mixed. Fold in the whipped cream, rosemary and salmon. Pour the mixture into individual soufflé dishes and allow to set in the refrigerator. Garnish each soufflé with red lumpfish roe before serving.

Herb and Cheese Soufflé

Serves: 4–5
1 1/4 cups (10 fl oz) milk
2 eggs, separated
125 g (4 oz) cheddar cheese, grated
90 g (3 oz) soft wholemeal breadcrumbs
1 tablespoon grated onion
1 tablespoon chopped parsley
2 teaspoons chopped tarragon
salt and pepper

Warm the milk and add it to the beaten egg yolks and other ingredients (except egg whites). Allow to stand for 1 hour. Whip the egg whites and fold in the mixture. Bake in a buttered ovenproof dish in a moderate oven (180°C/350°F/Gas 4) for 30 minutes.

An excellent, simply prepared luncheon or supper dish.

Garlic Rice with Crisp Fennel Stems

Serves 6-8
2½ cups (20 fl oz) water
pinch of salt
1 cup (5 oz) brown rice
1-2 teaspoons finely chopped garlic
1 fennel base or 'bulb', sliced thinly
*   and chopped*
2 teaspoons finely chopped fennel leaves
extra salt and freshly ground pepper

Bring the water to the boil in a saucepan, add a pinch of salt and the rice (wash only if dusty). Put the lid on and simmer gently until the water has been absorbed – about 40 minutes. If necessary place on a flame-proof mat to prevent the rice from sticking. Since the absorption rate of rice varies, more boiling water may need to be added – a little at a time – if the grains are still hard. When the rice is cooked, and dry, with a fork stir in the garlic and the chopped fennel base and leaves. Add salt and pepper to taste. Serve hot as a vegetable or cold as a salad.

To make a rice salad, let the rice cool, transfer to a bowl, cover with plastic film and chill. Before serving, toss the rice in a French dressing of 3 tablespoons oil to 1 tablespoon herb or wine vinegar. If a larger amount of dressing is preferred, increase the quantities of oil and vinegar, keeping the ratio of 3 to 1.
N.B. As brown rice is said to help reduce high blood-pressure, do not add salt and pepper to this recipe if you suffer from this complaint; include some very finely chopped young borage leaves (natural salt) instead, and some finely cut peppery winter savory.

Steamed Lemongrass Chicken

Serves 4
1 kg (2 lb) chicken
1¼ cups (10 fl oz) water
1 teaspoon salt
pinch of pepper
6-8 lemongrass leaves, coarsely chopped
1 tablespoon cornflour (cornstarch)
milk to mix

Place the chicken on a heavy saucer in a saucepan. Add the water, sprinkle the salt and pepper over the chicken and heap the lemongrass onto the breast. Put the lid on the saucepan, bring the water to the boil, then lower the heat and simmer for 2 hours, occasionally basting the chicken with the liquor in the saucepan. If the water is evaporating too quickly, place a flame-proof mat under the saucepan.

If the chicken is to be eaten hot, remove it to a serving dish and keep hot. Strain the stock into a small saucepan and add 1 tablespoon cornflour blended to a smooth paste with a little milk. Pour the thickened sauce over the chicken and serve.

If the chicken is to be eaten cold, put it into a deep bowl or dish and pour the strained stock over it. Cool, then cover and chill overnight. Next day, the stock will have jellied and a surface layer of fat will have formed which should be removed. The chicken will be aromatic and succulent.

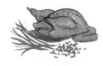

Gretta Anna's Potato Fans with Oregano, Cheese and Bacon

Serves 6

This recipe was given to use by a kind and close friend.

Take 6 medium potatoes all the same size. Peel and cut away a thin horizontal slice from the bottom of each, so that they will all sit flat. Slice each potato downwards all along in 3 mm (⅛ inch) slices, but do not cut right through to the base. Place potatoes in a roasting pan. Sprinkle the slit potatoes with salt, pepper, 1 tablespoon fresh, chopped oregano (or 3 teaspoons dried oregano), 6 teaspoons grated cheese and 6 teaspoons finely chopped bacon.

Roast the potatoes in a little oil to barely cover the bottom of the pan in a moderate oven 180°C (350°F/Gas 4) for approximately 1¼ hours or until golden-brown and cooked through. (Test with a skewer.) Roast potatoes flavoured and adorned like this are unusual and delicious.

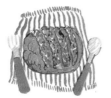

Cauliflower Cheese Teplitzky

Serves 6-8

This recipe is dedicated to Gretta Anna (a well-loved, inventive cook with tremendous flair) and her husband, David Teplitzky, their daughter Anna, and Gretta's ageless and enchanting mother, Mrs Schneideman. Sunday evening is a special time for us all to relax together and enjoy a simple but tasty meal, and these dear friends say that this is their favourite cauliflower cheese. The original recipe was my late, wonderful, mother's. We serve this fairly substantial dish with cold meat and mustard, a tossed green salad and hot herb bread, followed by fresh fruit.

1 medium to large cauliflower, cooked whole in salted water until just soft (test the stalk with a skewer, it should be crisp, but cooked)
4 cups (1 litre) béchamel sauce (not too thin)
2 tablespoons chopped parsley
1 tablespoon chopped chives
½ tablespoon chopped dill or chervil
1 cup (4 oz) grated melting cheese (Gruyère, or similar)
1 cup (4 oz) dry breadcrumbs

Turn the whole, cooked cauliflower into a colander to drain. Transfer to a fairly deep, buttered, ovenproof dish, flower-side up. Mix the herbs into the sauce and coat the cauliflower with it, letting the excess run into the dish. Mix the cheese and breadcrumbs and sprinkle them over the cauliflower. Put the dish into a moderate oven (180°C/350°F/Gas 4) for approximately 30-45 minutes until the cheese has melted and the cauliflower is hot. If the cheese begins to burn, cover with a piece of brown paper, or foil.

Spinach Fettuccine with Basil and Garlic

Serves 4-6

375 g (12 oz) spinach fettuccine (spinach spaghetti or plain spaghetti may be used instead)
125 g (4 oz) unsalted butter
2 cloves garlic, pounded, or very thinly sliced
1/2 cup (4 fl oz) thin cream
2 tablespoons freshly chopped basil (or 1 tablespoon dried basil: fresh or dried oregano may be substituted in the same proportions)
1/2 cup (2 oz) grated Parmesan cheese
pepper to taste

Boil a quantity of salted water in a large saucepan. Add fettuccine unbroken, gradually loosening it with a fork as it softens. Cook briskly, uncovered, for approximately 12-15 minutes until tender. Drain in a colander and immediately pour boiling water over the pasta, continuing to let it drain.

Meanwhile, melt butter, sauté garlic in it over a low heat, do not let it brown. Pour this mixture into a bowl and beat in the cream and basil. Now transfer the drained fettuccine into a warmed serving bowl and pour the butter and cream mixture over it with half the Parmesan cheese. Toss well with a spoon and fork, adding extra cheese gradually while doing this and seasoning with the pepper – freshly ground if possible.

Before bringing to the table sprinkle more grated Parmesan over the cooked fettuccine. Garnish with a few sprigs of fresh basil or oregano (optional). Serve hot with crusty bread and a tossed crisp salad. A bowl of Parmesan should be handed around at the table in case more is needed to sprinkle over the vanishing portions of this fragrant and deliciously soothing dish.

Rice and Herb Spinach Rolls

Serves: 4–6

12 young spinach leaves
1 cup (5 oz) uncooked rice
1 onion, finely chopped
1/2 capsicum (green pepper), seeded and chopped
1 tablespoon chopped parsley
1 teaspoon each of 2 or 3 other favourite herbs, chopped: e.g., marjoram, chervil, tarragon and bergamot, or sage, dill, oregano and rosemary
salt and pepper (lemon pepper preferably)
2 chicken stock cubes dissolved in 1 1/2 cups (12 fl oz) hot water, or an equivalent amount of stock

Wash spinach leaves and trim off stalk edges. Mix together the rice, onion, capsicum, herbs, salt and pepper. Place 1 tablespoon of rice mixture on each flattened spinach leaf, and roll into neat envelope shapes. Pack into a saucepan. Pour the stock over the rolls. Place a weight over the rolls (a dessert plate will do), and put the lid on the saucepan. Bring the stock to the boil, turn down the heat and simmer for 45 minutes.

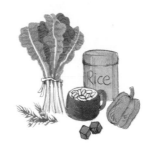

Steak and Kidney Casserole

Serves 4-6
500 g (1 lb) steak and kidney, chopped
*   and mixed*
3 tablespoons flour
2 large cloves garlic, chopped
1 small onion, chopped
2 medium-sized carrots, chopped
1 outside stalk celery, chopped
2 teaspoons salt
freshly ground pepper
A fresh bouquet garni, made with a stalk
*   of bay leaves, a spray each of parsley,*
*   marjoram and thyme tied together with a*
*   long piece of string, or*
2 teaspoons dried, crumbled bouquet
*   garni*
1¼ cups (10 fl oz) water or stock

Preheat the oven to 180°C (350°F/Gas 4). Roll the meat in the flour and put into an ovenproof casserole dish with the rest of the ingredients, add the water last. Put the lid on and place in the oven for about 2 hours. (Stir once or twice during this time.) Remove the fresh *bouquet garni* by pulling out the piece of string holding it together – the stalks will be mostly skeletal by this time, the leaves having floated into the gravy. Serve hot.

Steaming herb dumplings are delicious with this casserole, and should be dropped onto the bubbling mixture 20 minutes before the end of the cooking time.

Herb Dumplings

Sift 1 cup (4 oz) self-raising flour into a bowl, add half a teaspoon of salt and rub in 40 g (1½ oz) butter or margarine. Add a tablespoon of chopped parsley, marjoram or oregano and enough cold water to make a stiff dough. Rub flour onto your hands and form the dough into balls; add them to the casserole. Do not replace the lid. Cook for 20 minutes.

Braised Chicory With Dill

Serves: 4
500 g (1 lb) chicory heads
1 tablespoon chopped chives
2 teaspoons chopped green dill (or chervil,
fennel, or oregano)
butter or vegetable margarine
salt and pepper

Wash and trim the chicory. Cut into thick circles and pack into a buttered ovenproof dish with the herbs, salt, pepper and pieces of butter between each layer. Put the lid on and bake in a moderate oven (180°C/350°F/Gas 4) for 1¼ to 1½ hours.
N.B. The chicory must be of the best quality, the leaves white, without any trace of green. If you like, the heads can be boiled in water first for a few minutes to help remove any bitterness.

Oregano and Capsicum Relish

3 red capsicums (red peppers)
3 green capsicums (green peppers)
2 onions, peeled and chopped
2 cloves garlic, peeled and chopped finely
1 cup (8 fl oz) white wine vinegar
1 cup (8 oz) raw sugar
2 teaspoons salt
1 tablespoon chopped fresh oregano leaves
2 tablespoons seedless raisins

Wash the capsicums, cut into small pieces, discarding the seeds. Put all the ingredients together in a saucepan and bring to the boil, then simmer with the lid off for 1 hour. Seal into jars when cold. Refrigerate once the jar is opened.

Cucumber and Green Herb Sauce

1 cucumber, peeled, seeded and diced
salt
1 small bunch seedless grapes, picked from their stalks
1 tablespoon parsley or chervil, finely chopped
1 tablespoon chives, finely chopped
2 teaspoons spearmint, finely chopped
1 cup low fat sour cream
pinch of ground chilli or a little pepper

Mix all ingredients together in a bowl. Chill. Serve with curries, or put on a buffet table as an accompaniment to other dishes.

Pestou

Pestou is an excellent way to preserve and freeze basil. Use it as a spread, or fold it through freshly cooked, drained pasta. This is Mrs Clare Wilmot's recipe, which first appeared in *Herbs, Their Cultivation and Usage* by John and Rosemary Hemphill, published by Lansdowne Press.

1 large bunch of sweet basil, or a smaller bunch of bush basil
125 g (4 oz) grated Parmesan cheese
125 g (4 oz) pine kernels
4 cloves garlic, peeled
a little sea salt
cold pressed oil

Wash the basil and strip the leaves from the stems. Place all the ingredients in a blender, with a little oil. Turn the blender to high, adding more oil if necessary, until the ingredients are pulverised. The mixture should have the consistency of thick, running cream. Use immediately, or store, covered, in the refrigerator, or seal down in small jars and deep-freeze.

Mango-Cream with Angelica

My mother's recipe for this fragrant, smooth dessert, reminds me of school holidays spent long ago in Broome, about 2000 km from Perth, in Western Australia, where my brother and I were at boarding school. We used to go home by ship once in every twelve months for the eight-week Christmas vacation and Fred and I always invited a school-friend so that they could experience a different Australia, and we could repay kindness shown to us during the year. A week's cruising in a small but immaculate Blue Funnel Line steamer with other youngsters going home to various stops along the desolate north-west coast, and to Java, Singapore, Malaya and Hong Kong, was always fun, even though we sometimes struck frighteningly rough seas, and once the edge of a cyclone when the Captain put on full speed to race away from it, while the ship pitched and rolled like a cork, and we slithered, climbed, and ran down heaving decks.

At dinner in Broome, our Mango-Cream was served in chilled glasses as we sat around the massive teak table, made by Father's Japanese carpenter (who also helped build his pearling luggers), under a whirring ceiling fan to stir the hot air, and to prevent platoons of moths and thin, jade-green grasshoppers from falling into the food. Outside, the sheet lightning flickered constantly, the vast colonies of cicadas who shrilled during the intense day-time heat gave occasional chirps, the warm breeze rustled the long pandanus leaves by the door, and the Aborigines in their camp nearby clicked ceremonial sticks, or danced their corroborees. Every noise was audible since we were surrounded by spacious verandahs enclosed only by low, latticed wooden rails and huge, half-open, flat-iron "shutters" that were fastened down when violent "cock-eye-bobs", or fierce cyclones, struck. The iron roof was anchored securely to the ground by steel cables to stop the house from blowing away in a bad storm. Houses were built on top of high cement blocks for coolness, and to prevent white ants from eating the house down, as well as to deter snakes and scorpions from entering, which they did at times anyway. The stars there in The Tropic of Capricorn were closer and more plentiful, their incandescent brilliance lighting the sky to indigo; and every night falling stars plunged blazing towards us, only to disappear into the galaxy again.

To make her Mango-Cream, Mother had access to superb mangoes of several flavours, which Father and the Aboriginal, Tommy, grew with pride, in between sorties for pearls at sea. Fresh cream was out of the question, the cow's milk, when available, was thin and poor because of lack of good feed in that red, arid soil: instead, nearly every family kept at least one goat for its nourishing milk. Our mother, a typical "English rose", had never been inside a kitchen before she went to Broome, but she gamely made the best of things and relied on Nestlé's canned cream and imported angelica. Of course there were no blenders in those days, so she used to laboriously squeeze all the juice from the flesh around the mango stones, after having sliced the rest of the flesh off and pulped it, and the canned cream was not whipped. Tora, the Japanese cook, our beloved childhood friend, was never allowed to make this dish, for it was Mother's speciality. Fresh cream is used in this adaptation.

Serves 6-8
2 tablespoons gelatine
4 tablespoons very hot water
4-6 fresh mangoes, peeled and cut away from the seed, or
2 cans mango purée, or sliced mango puréed in the blender
2 tablespoons sifted icing (confectioner's) sugar (or icing sugar mixture)
2 tablespoons rum or liqueur
1¼ cups (10 fl oz) cream, whipped
extra whipped cream for decorating
candied angelica stalks, or crystallised mint leaves

Dissolve the gelatine in the hot water and stir until clear. Put all the ingredients into a blender, except the whipped cream and angelica or crystallised mint. Turn to high until the mixture is amalgamated. (This may have to be done in batches, depending on the size of the blender.) Pour the mixture into a bowl and fold in the whipped cream. Spoon into individual glasses or silver goblets, or into one attractive bowl. Chill until set. Before serving, decorate with the extra whipped cream and sticks of candied angelica. If you do not have candied angelica or crystallised mint leaves, use fresh mint sprigs instead.

N.B. Puréed fresh guavas, or canned guavas puréed in a blender, may be used instead of the mangoes for a change.

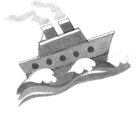

Strawberry Cream

Several years in Kentish England spent with maternal grandparents during part of our childhood seemed like living in a heaven of vivid, yet gentle, greens; softly glowing flowers with pure, lingering fragrances; musical bird calls; different tastes of fruit and vegetables, and a life where all was ordered, calm and gracious. (Such a contrast to Australia's semi-tropical Broome with its simmering heat, surreal landscapes, shrilling cicadas, raucous parrots, and the overpowering, sickly sweet scent of oleander flowers.) The secluded garden, with its velvet lawns, was large, beautiful, and very English – (no Italianate influences here). Much of it was 200 years old and included a particularly venerable oak tree. The many walks and hidden places were a paradise for children to play in. There were the oak and horse-chestnut trees to climb (and a warning not to clamber up ancient yew trees, which left black marks on clothes). At first we trod cautiously through the long grass in the orchard for fear of lurking snakes, which greatly amused our mother, grandparents, uncles and aunts. "Not here, darling," they would say.

An ivy-cloaked, brick-walled garden, intersected by a stone-arched doorway, beckoned to another part of this fascinating Eden, where there was the kitchen garden with fruit and vegetables grown for the house. In late spring and summer there was an abundance of strawberries, redcurrants, blackcurrants, whitecurrants, raspberries, gooseberries, asparagus, baby new potatoes and other vegetables. Sun-warmed peaches and nectarines were plucked only by Grandfather from fruit trees espaliered against one side of the wall. In this sequestered garden, huge pink roses annually twined their way along ropes; and one dense, green, rose bush bore masses of small white blooms more exquisitely perfumed than any other flower. It was truly an enchanted garden and, sadly, no longer exists. Rows of new houses now take its place and the old trees have gone too.

Sunday trifles were a treat; whipped cream was spread over this favourite pudding and it was strewn with candied violets and pink rose petals (see page 102 for how to crystallise flowers and leaves), silver cachous glistening among them. Strawberry cream garnished with crystallised mint leaves was another glorious flavour feast never forgotten. This is how it was made, at the peak of the strawberry season:

Grandmother's Strawberry Cream

Serves: about 10, depending on the amount of cream and strawberries used
thickened cream
ripe strawberries, hulled
caster (powdered) sugar
crystallised mint leaves (page 102)

Chill a deep bowl and half fill it with cream. Whip the cream lightly, then put into it as many strawberries as possible, mashing them gently with a fork while doing so. (Cut large berries in half and put small ones in whole.) When the cream is saturated with strawberries, put the mixture into a serving bowl, smooth the top of the Strawberry Cream and chill it for at least an hour in the refrigerator. Before serving, sift some castor sugar over the top and decorate with crystallised mint leaves. (Blackberries, loganberries, raspberries and boysenberries may be used instead of the strawberries.)

French Chocolate Mousse Garnished with Crystallised Violets

Serves 4
The quantities can be doubled to serve 8, or tripled to serve 12.

60 g (2 oz) dark cooking chocolate
40 g (1½ oz) unsalted (sweet) butter
3 eggs, separated
4 tablespoons caster (powdered) sugar
1 tablespoon rum
whipped cream for decorating, and crystallised violets, rose petals or mint leaves

Melt the chocolate and butter in the top of a double saucepan, stirring occasionally, until very smooth. (Alternatively, stand a bowl (not plastic) in a saucepan of simmering water.)

Beat the egg yolks and sugar together, then add to the chocolate, stirring until smooth.

Remove from the stove and whisk in the rum. Beat the egg whites until stiff and fold them into the chocolate mixture. Pour into individual dishes, or a serving bowl. Chill in the refrigerator until firm. Decorate with the whipped cream and the crystallised flowers or leaves.

Marmalade of Violets

Half a pound [250 g] of violet flowers, one and a half pounds of sugar [750 g], half a cup of water.

Take half a pound of violet flowers picked from their stalks and crush them in a mortar.

Boil the sugar and water to a syrup, and when boiling add the flowers. Allow it to come five or six times to the boil on a very slow fire. Stir it with a wooden spoon, and pour it while hot into little pots.

Lemon and Balm Soufflé

Serves 6
2 tablespoons gelatine
8 tablespoons very hot water
6 eggs, separated
375 g (12 oz) caster (powdered) sugar
grated rind and strained juice of 4 lemons
1 tablespoon very finely chopped balm leaves
1¼ cups (10 fl oz) cream, whipped

Dissolve the gelatine in the hot water; stir with a spoon until clear. Beat the sugar thoroughly into the egg yolks and then gradually beat in the rind and juice of the lemons and add the balm leaves. Put the egg yolk mixture in a double saucepan and whisk over gentle heat until thick and creamy. Remove from the heat and beat a little longer. Whip the egg whites until they stand in peaks. Add the dissolved gelatine to the lemon mixture and fold in the whipped egg whites and cream. Spoon into a serving dish and set in the refrigerator.

Ice Cream of Roses

One pint cream [2½s cups or 20 fl oz or 620 ml], two handfuls of fresh rose petals, yolks of two eggs, sugar.

Boil a pint of cream and put into it when it boils two handfuls of fresh rose petals, and leave them for two hours, well covered. Then pass this through a sieve, and mix with the cream the well-beaten yolks of two eggs, and sugar to taste. Add a little cochineal, and put it on the fire, stirring it all the time, but do not let it boil on any account. Put it on ice.

Salads with herbs and edible flowers

Green salads that are generously laced with aromatic herbs have an appealing relish and help to stimulate the appetite, as well as being packed with health-giving properties. Some of the lesser known "salad greens" to use as a base include mignonette lettuce, cos lettuce, chicory or witloof, celery tops, torn up leaves of English spinach (not as coarse as silver beet), finely sliced heads of raw young cabbage, and young cauliflowers. If you don't grow these yourself, they are readily available from most greengrocers.

Green dill finely cut and mixed into a coleslaw with a few dill seeds makes the cabbage more digestible, and imparts its subtle anise flavour.

Quantities of fresh parsley and mint, chopped finely, are included in that nutritious and delectable Lebanese salad, Tabbouleh.

Borage leaves add a natural, salty flavour to salads, and the brilliant blue flowers are edible too. Because of the hairy texture of the leaves, they should be very finely chopped, almost minced.

Nasturtium leaves are often added to salads and sandwiches. Their keen, hot taste makes them a useful replacement for pepper in many dishes. Pick young, tender leaves and eat them whole in salads: put a cluster of jewel-coloured flowers in the middle of a Salad Nicoise, and eat them too.

Fresh winter and summer savory can be used instead of pepper in salads.

Basil, bergamot, cress, chervil, chives, tarragon, fennel, mint, balm, comfrey, angelica, lovage, small quantities of coriander, marjoram, oregano, finely chopped fresh rosemary and sage, are excellent herbs to mix into a green salad; they all grow through summer, into autumn, and some even later. There are numerous wild plants you can use in salads, including chickweed and dandelion leaves, so when you are weeding, don't dig them all up, keep some for the kitchen. Of course, not all weeds are edible, so if in doubt do not eat them.

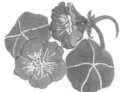

A flower salad

A "flower" salad doesn't necessarily have to be made from flowers, it can be made from many ingredients, but because of the way it is arranged it looks like one large flower, and tastes quite heavenly. It has been said that: "In eating flowers we partake of the more refined essences of the plant, the final stage before returning to seed and completing the circle of plant life. So the flower offers a more subtle energy, as well as sweet nectar... flowers can speak to us and contain special healing powers. To gather and make this salad is one way of being with flowers and learning how they express the harmony of nature." *(Jeanne Rose's Herbal Guide to Inner Health* published by Grosset and Dunlap, New York.) Not all flowers are edible, so make sure the ones you choose *are*.

To make a flower salad, you will need a flat, large, round china or glass platter, or a round tray. On it make a bed of some of the larger herb leaves, for instance angelica, lovage, comfrey, nasturtium, chicory or dandelion. In the centre put a mound of grated carrot, and circle it with small, broken sprigs of washed, raw young cauliflower florets. Next, make a circle of colourful nasturtium flowers interspersed with honeyed bergamot flowers and leaf sprigs, then a surround of alfalfa, or any other favourite sprouts. Around this, make a rainbow circle of sky-blue borage flowers, purple violets, pink or red rose petals, and yellow stars of dill or fennel flowers. Surround the plate with sprays of curly parsley and spearmint tops. If there is still room, add radish "roses" and crisp curled celery to the flowery platter. Pour a light dressing over all before bearing it to the table. This salad may be made an hour ahead of time and kept fresh in the refrigerator, but do not add the dressing until the very last moment.

Light Salad Dressing – Put 6 tablespoons of a fine salad oil (walnut or hazelnut oil) into a clean bottle or jar with a lid, add 2 tablespoons of herb or wine vinegar (or lemon juice), salt, freshly ground pepper, and a small teaspoon of clear honey. Put the lid on, shake well, and pour a sufficient amount over the salad without drowning it. Store any leftover dressing in the refrigerator.

Green herb salad

Quantities are your choice

spearmint leaves stripped from their
  stalks
watercress leaves
cos lettuce
chives, finely chopped
chickweed
young dandelion leaves

Wash and thoroughly dry all the ingredients. Tear up the larger leaves, and put all the greens together in a salad bowl. Cover with plastic film and crisp in the refrigerator for a few hours, or overnight. Before serving, pour on some Light Salad Dressing and toss well.

Herbed potato and banana salad

3 cups diced, peeled, cooked potatoes
  (boiled in their skins and peeled
  while warm)
1 cup sliced banana
a little fresh lemon or lime juice
salt and pepper
1 cup finely chopped spring onions
  (scallions), including the green part
1 tablespoon either chopped basil,
  dill, tarragon or chervil
1 cup (8 fl oz) mayonnaise
2 hard-boiled eggs, shelled and sliced

Sprinkle lemon or lime juice over the banana slices to prevent discoloration. While the potatoes are still warm, season them with salt and pepper and add the banana and spring onions. Blend the chopped herbs with the mayonnaise and mix gently through the salad. Add the egg slices. Chill before serving.

Salad Marie Louise

Take equal parts of sliced boiled cold potatoes and raw peeled and sliced apples. Add oil, salt and pepper. Mix at the last moment and place in a mound in the centre of the salad bowl. Sprinkle with crushed hard-boiled eggs. Surround with alternative small mounds of corn and of violets, stems removed. (Alice B. Toklas, *Aromas and Flavors*, 1958.)

Green Lima Bean and Basil Salad

Serves: 4

This salad may be flavoured with any one of your favourite herbs. Choose either basil, as suggested above or, if it is out of season, oregano, marjoram, rosemary, mint, tarragon, dill, chervil, or fennel. A discreet amount of chopped fresh coriander leaves gives the salad an unusual and piquant flavour.

2 cups (1 lb) frozen or canned small green lima beans
1 tablespoon finely chopped basil
2 shallots (spring onions), finely chopped
salt and pepper
4 tablespoons vegetable, or walnut, or hazel nut oil blended with 1 tablespoon white vinegar or lemon juice

Boil the frozen beans in salted water until cooked. If using canned beans, drain and rinse, then drain again. Put the beans into a bowl and add the basil, shallots, salt and pepper to taste, and the oil and vinegar mixture last. Toss well.

Chrysanthemum Salad

Clean and wash in several waters about twenty chrysanthemum flowers picked from the stalks. Blanch them in acidulated and salted water; drain them and dry them in a cloth.

Mix them well into a salad composed of potatoes, artichoke bottoms, shrimps' tails, and capers in vinegar.

Arrange this in a salad bowl, and decorate it with beetroot and hard-boiled egg. A pinch of saffron may be added to this salad for seasoning.

The dark yellow chrysanthemums are best. In Yokohama the flowers, already prepared, are sold in the greengrocers' shops.

The Gentle Art of Cookery, by Mrs C. F. Leyel and Miss Olga Hartley, published by Chatto & Windus.

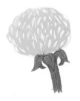

Elderflower Sorbet

Serves: 4–6
2½ cups (20 fl oz) water
185 g (6 oz) sugar
4 heads of fresh elderflowers
peeled rind and juice of 3 lemons
1 egg white, whipped

Put the water into a saucepan with the sugar. Heat until sugar is completely dissolved, stirring with a wooden spoon to prevent it sticking to the bottom. Boil rapidly, uncovered, for about 5 to 8 minutes and add the whole elderflowers. Turn off the heat and allow the flowers to infuse in the syrup for several minutes. Stir in the lemon rind and juice. Strain the syrup into a bowl, let it cool, then pour it into freezing trays and put into the freezer. When half frozen, turn it into a clean bowl and mix in the egg white, beating with a rotary beater to amalgamate the mixture. Put it back into the trays and freeze again. A sorbet becomes smoother with several beatings during the freezing process, although this is optional.

Serve this unusual and delicious ice either as a palate cleanser during a meal, or as a dessert.

Culpeper's Colour Herbal, David Potterton (ed.) (W. Foulsham, London, 1983).

Culpeper, Nicholas, *Culpeper's Complete Herbal* (W. Foulsham, London).

Geuter, Maria, *Herbs in Nutrition* (Bio-Dynamic Agricultural Association, London, 1962).

Rudolf Hauschka D.Sc., *Nutrition,* translated from the German by Marjoria Spock and Mary T. Richards (Stuart & Watkins, London, 1967).

Grieve, Mrs M., *A Modern Herbal,* 2 vols., Mrs C. F. Leyel (ed.) (Hafner Publishing Co., New York, 1959).

Hemphill, John and Rosemary, *Hemphill's Herbs, Their Cultivation and Usage* (Lansdowne Press, Sydney, 1983).

Lotions and Potions (compiled by the National Federation of Women's Institutes, England, 1956, Novello, London).

Rohde, Eleanour Sinclair, *A Garden of Herbs* (Medici Society, London).

Wilmot, Clare, *Triad Health Products,* Literature, from St. Ives, N.S.W.

The Coronation Cookery Book, compiled for The Country Women's Association of N.S.W., Australia, by Jessie Sawyer, O.B.E. and Sara-Moore-Sims, 1947.

Rohde, Eleanour Sinclair, *Shakespeare's Wild Flowers* (Medici Society, London, 1963).

Rose, Jeanne, *Jeanne Rose's Herbal Guide to Inner Health* (Grosset & Dunlap, New York, 1980).

The Holy Bible.

Law, Donald, *Herbal Teas for Health and Pleasure* (Health Science Press, England, 1968).

Father John Künzle, *Herbs and Weeds* (Salvioni & Co. S.A., Bellinzona, Switzerland, 1975).

The Encyclopedia of Herbs and Herbalism, Malcolm Stuart (ed.) (Paul Hamlyn, Sydney, 1979).

Hemphill, Rosemary, *The Penguin Book of Herbs and Spices* (Penguin Books, Harmondsworth, 1966).

Hemphill, Rosemary, *Herbs for All Seasons* (Angus & Robertson, Sydney, 1972).

Janssen, Sally, E. *Incense* (The Triad Library & Publishing Co., St. Ives, NSW, 1968).

Barnard, Julian, *Bach Flower Remedies* (The C.W. Daniel Co. Ltd, Essex, England, 1979).

Ross, Gordon A. C., *Homoeopathy* (Thorsons Publishers Ltd, Northamptonshire, 1976).

Ryman, Danièle, *The Aromatherapy Handbook* (Century Publishing Co. Ltd, 1984).

Rohde, E. S., *The Scented Garden* (The Medici Society, London).

Nature and Health magazine (RPLA Pty Ltd, Dee Why, Australia).

Harmsworth's Universal Encyclopedia (The Educational Book Co. Ltd, London).